ALL AMERICAN
Berries

ALL AMERICAN
Berries

Potent Foods for Lasting Health

Francis Brinker, N.D.

Eclectic Medical Publications
Sandy, Oregon

For permission to reproduce selections from this book,
write to:
Eclectic Medical Publications
12960 SE Ten Eyck
Sandy Oregon 97055
Printed in the USA

Production by Fourth Lloyd Productions, LLC
Book and Cover Design by Richard Stodart

ISBN: 978-1-888483-18-5 paperback
1-88848318-0 (10 digit number)

Library of Congress Control Number: 2015939398

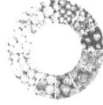

Dedication

To my Dad and Mom, Francis and Julia, for their love and faith and hard work growing and preparing the fruits, vegetables, grains, beans, chickens, pigs, sheep, and dairy cattle on our family farm to feed their children and others.

TABLE OF CONTENTS

Table of Contents (*cont'd*)

PREFACE

This book began as an Appendix to another text on indigenous American medicinal plants. It was intended to complement the information on botanical therapeutics with a brief consideration about the role of American berries in health and disease. As the content of the original book continued to grow, the Appendix likewise ballooned as more and more research accrued on the preventive and therapeutic value of certain American berries. Eventually, the scientific research on these berries and their significance to modern health concerns outgrew its initial context and became so compelling that the need for a separate book became obvious.

Health care providers in particular need to be aware of the evidence that is available on the specific benefits of common food items. As the quality and quantity of research on the value of these and other berries continues to expand, this text serves as an alert to the importance of including these powerful foods as regular components in our diets. Given the degenerative health issues of our aging populations and the need to protect healthy tissues and cellular functions from the insidious damage that occurs from long-term oxidative stress, the most practical means of lowering the risk of developing associated chronic disease conditions is ingestion of the most healthful vegetables and fruits, especially berries.

Since the challenge of eating an optimal diet has always left some well-intentioned consumers in its wake, the availability of concentrated berry products such as dehydrated powders and extracts helps make intake of the potent berry components easier. Unfortunately, many forms of preparations, including commercial juices and canned products, usually contain significant amounts of sugars that undermine much of the health-promoting value. The choices made to accommodate personal preferences should be well informed to best suit individual needs. This book provides compelling evidence for those wanting to improve their own and/or their patients' current and future health through easy and effective dietary means.

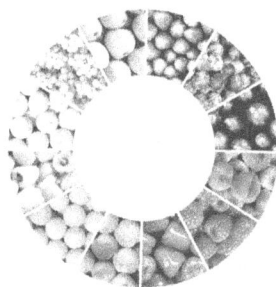

ONE

WHOLE FRUITS AND VEGETABLES FOR HELPING PREVENT CHRONIC DISEASES

THERE IS CONSENSUS AMONG THE SCIENTIFIC AND HEALTHCARE COMMUNITY THAT THE CONSUMPTION OF A WHOLE-FOOD, PLANT-BASED DIET PROVIDES THE BEST PROTECTION AGAINST DEVELOPING MANY CHRONIC DISEASES. THE DISEASE-PREVENTION VALUE OF EATING WHOLE GRAINS, BEANS, NUTS, AND ESPECIALLY VEGETABLES AND FRUITS IS BASED NOT ONLY ON THEIR CONTENT OF ESSENTIAL NUTRIENTS, THOUGH TOGETHER THEY ARE SUPERB SOURCES OF CARBOHYDRATES, PROTEINS, FATS, VITAMINS, AND MINERALS. THE COLORFUL ARRAY OF BOTANICAL CAROTENES AND "SECONDARY" POLYPHENOLIC COMPOUNDS HELP PROTECT AGAINST OXIDATIVE STRESS AND, TOGETHER WITH THE FIBER THAT PACKAGES THE PHYTOCHEMICAL MATRIX, ARE OF MAJOR IMPORTANCE FOR OPTIMIZING HEALTH. WITH BERRIES, THESE AND OTHER CONTRIBUTORS TO ANTI-INFLAMMATORY BIOACTIVITY COMBINE TO SUPPLY A WEALTH OF DIETARY TREASURE.

When a particular nutrient is shown by medical research to improve health or to prevent or ameliorate some disease condition, the public is invariably urged to consume foods that are high in that component rather than simply taking it supplementally as an isolated compound. This is certainly good advice regarding disease prevention, though isolated nutrients, similar to isolated drug components from plants, can be therapeutic for individuals with needs that manifest as deficiency symptoms or in conditions with exaggerated requirements. In regard to the prevention of cardiovascular diseases, the American Heart Association appropriately advocates the superiority of eating whole fruit and vegetables over the consumption of juices.

On the whole, fruit and vegetables contain a complex array of bioactive nutrient and fiber components that work together, rather than isolates acting individually. There is a growing awareness in the medical community about the importance of plant components and metabolites that function as semi-essential nutrients.[1] These compounds are seen as a rainbow of colors in our diet, often having antioxidant and free radical scavenging properties. They coexist as important components of medicinal and culinary herbs, spices, vegetables, fruit, and berries. Without an adequate supply of these adjunctive plant compounds, tissue deterioration may not be as dramatic or rapid as in the absence of required vitamins and minerals, yet still, these bioactive phytochemicals are an integral part of the design of nature. They help to facilitate protective biological processes and optimal physiological function, and so act to maintain and prolong good health in humans.

Plants of the Americas are invaluable contributors to the world's food riches. Vegetables originating here have become integral parts of intercontinental cuisine, in some cases becoming even more closely associated with countries on other continents than our own. For example, edible members of the nightshade family (Solanaceae) include the South American potato, the Mesoamerican green and red peppers (*Capsicum* spp.), and tomatoes (*Lycopersicon esculentum*). In addition, corn (*Zea mays*), beans (*Phaseolis vulgaris*), and squash (*Cucurbita* spp.), known as the "three sisters", were staples of the Central and North American native diet. In this context, the value of native North American berries will be emphasized here.

COLORS OF HEALTH

Pigments giving color to herbs, roots, flowers, and fruits are part of a complex chemical matrix in plants that can be additive, complementary, and/or synergistic in their physiological effects. Chlorophyll, the leaf pigment *par excellence* that makes plants green, captures radiant solar energy for conversion to energy stored as sugars. The transition of energy forms generates charges and free radicals that would create havoc from oxidative damage were it not for the protective antioxidants also produced to prevent this.

Carotenes, the yellow, orange, or red isomers common in vegetables, are exemplary in delivering antioxidant protection to plants and people. Of course, carrots are famous for supplying the aptly-named alpha- and beta-carotene. Dark green vegetables like kale and spinach also provide beta-carotene plus the xanthophyll (Greek for yellow leaf) carotenoids lutein and zeaxanthin in substantial amounts. The red carotene called lycopene found in tomatoes and watermellon is thus available from the garden as either a tangy or sweet juicy treat. For disease prevention, foods containing beta-carotene or lycopene appear to help reduce cancer risk, while those with lutein and zeaxanthin may help protect the eyes from macular degeneration.[2]

These 5 carotenoids, along with beta-cryptoxanthin, were examined for their dietary impact on metabolic syndrome prevalence in 374 middle-aged and older men. Total carotenoid, beta-carotene, and lycopene intake were significantly associated with a reduced risk of metabolic syndrome, while these 3 factors and alpha-carotene were all related to lower visceral fat, subcutaneous fat, and waist circumerfences. Higher lycopene intake was also associated with lower serum triglycerides.[3]

Along with chlorophyll and carotenes, fruit and vegetable colors can be due to various polyphenolics that have distinctive bioactivity.[4] Polyphenols are often responsible for the various hues that make plant flowers and fruits so attractive. The red, blue, and deep purple anthocyanin (*anthos* is Greek for flower and *cyanos* is Greek for blue) pigments are typically found in greatest concentrations and diversity in flowers and berries. Many of the native American berries are members the genera *Vaccinium* (e.g., cranberries, blueberries, and huckleberries) and *Rubus* (e.g., blackberries, red raspberries, black raspberries).[1] The anthocyanin and other phenolic compounds in these berries vary from species to species and even within different commercial cultivars of a single species. However, often one berry species will share many of the same components with other species of the same genus. For example, besides similar anthocyanins, *Vaccinium* species berries contain proanthocyanidins in common, whereas berries of *Rubus* species share ellagitannins. Both of these types of polyphenols serve as potent antioxidants.[1,5,6]

The red, blue, and deep purple anthocyanin
(*anthos* is Greek for flower and *cyanos* is Greek
for blue) pigments are typically found in greatest
concentrations and diversity in flowers and berries.[1]

Common polyphenols in berries are categorized as phenolic acids (e.g., gallic acid and ellagic acid) and flavonoids. Flavonoids are typically yellow, as their name implies (*flavus* is Latin for yellow), and are found in both fruit and vegetables. Flavonoids are often attached to a sugar molecule, such as glucose, to form flavonoid glycosides. This form enhances the water solubility of flavonoids and also can improve their absorption from the intestines into the bloodstream.[4] Flavonoids include flavanols (e.g., catechin, epicatechin), flavanones (e.g., hesperetin, naringenin), flavonols (e.g., quercetin, myricetin, kaempferol), flavones (e.g., apigenin, luteolin), and anthocyanidins (e.g., cyanidin, delphinidin). Flavanol polymers such as oligomeric proanthocyanidins are condensed tannins, while hydrolyzable tannins have a central sugar bound to several phenolic acid derivatives as in ellagitannins and gallotannins.[1,4,7] These dietary flavonoids work through a variety of mechanism to attenuate and prevent inflammation as potential neuroprotective, cardioprotective, and chemopreventive phytochemicals.[7]

The flavonols myricetin, quercetin, and quercetin glycosides are particularly abundant in *Vaccinium* species, whereas quercetin glycosides were predominant in *Rubus* and *Aronia* species.[8,9] These flavonoids are greatly reduced during processing, as shown with total quercetin and kaempferol contents in fresh *Vaccinium* and *Rubus* species versus their jams.[10] Likewise, on a dry weight basis, fresh berries such as cranberries contain a much greater total polyphenol content than dried fruit. Still, the dried fruit provides greater antioxidant activity than isolated vitamins C, E, or beta-carotene.[11] In a study of the preservation in strawberries of color, total anthocyanins, total polyphenols, and vitamin C, freeze-drying was shown to be superior to convection drying, vacuum drying, and vacuum-microwave drying. The antioxidant activity of freeze-dried strawberries, as measured by several methods, was as good or better than for berries that underwent vacuum-microwave drying and superior to the convection or vaccum-dried berries.[12]

Reducing Risks of Cardiovascular Disease and Cancer

The beneficial outcomes of polyphenolic antioxidant activity are far-ranging when the impact on chronic degenerative diseases is considered. In Americans free from cancer, diabetes and cardiovascular disease at baseline, 70,359 women in the first Nurses Health Study (NHS) from 1984-2008 and 89,201 in the second NHS (NHS II) from 1991-2007, together with 41,334 men in the Health Professionals Follow-up Study (HPFS) from 1986-2006 were assessed base on food-frequency questionnaires. Among these, 12,611 cases of type 2 diabetes developed. A lower risk of type 2 diabetes was significantly associated with higher anthocyanin intake, especially from eating blueberries more than twice weekly compared to less than once per month and pooled consumption of apples/pears eaten at least 5 times per week versus less than once monthly.[13]

A lower risk of type 2 diabetes was significantly associated with higher anthocyanin intake.[13]

In general, consumption of flavonoids from berries has been shown to reduce biomarkers associated with metabolic syndrome.[14] In looking at women in NHS I and NHS II, and men in HPFS who were cancer-free and without stroke, heart disease, high blood pressure or treatment for hypertension, after 14 years of follow-up 5629 cases of hypertension in men and 29,018 cases in women were reported. A multivariate-adjusted analysis found that the 20% who consumed the highest quantities (top quintile) of anthocyanins (mostly blueberries and strawberries) had an 8% significantly reduced risk of having high blood pressure, compared to the lowest 20% of anthocyanin intake. The risk reduction was even greater, over 12%, for those of ages 60 years or less. A 5% reduced risk was also found for the flavone apigenin, and a 5-7% reduction in those 60 years or less for the flavanols epicatechin and catechin, when comparing the highest 20% and lowest 20% of consumption of these flavonoids.[15]

Prospective cohort studies, such as the NHS with 75,596 women from ages 34 to 59 years with 14 years follow-up and the HPFS with 38,683 men from ages 40 to 75 years with 8 years of follow-up, looked at the risk of ischemic stroke in the context of fruit and vegetable intake. All were free of cardiovascular disease, diabetes, and cancer at baseline. Those persons in the highest 20% of fruit and vegetable intake had a median of 5.8 and 5.1 servings daily among the women and men, respectively; these had a relative risk of 0.69 (about 2/3 of the risk of stroke), compared to those 20% with the lowest intake. Each increment of 1 serving daily was associated with a 6% lower risk of ischemic stroke.[16]

In 2013 a follow-up on the NHS II, involving 93,600 women between the ages of 25 and 42 years who were healthy at the 1989 baseline, examined the relationship between the risk of myocardial infarction (MI), commonly referred to as a heart attack, and the consumption of anthocyanins and other types of flavonoids. Updated and validated food-frequency questionnaires, collected every 4 years and used to estimate intakes of categories of flavonoids, indicated a significant inverse relationship between higher anthocyanin intake and risk of MI after multivariate adjustment. Other flavonoids did not show a significant relationship. The combined intake of blueberries and strawberries greater than 3 times weekly tended to be associated with a lower MI risk, compared to those who consumed these less frequently.[17]

In the prospective Iowa Women's Health Study of almost 34,500 postmenopausal women over a 16 year period, the consumption of total flavonoids of different classes were found to correlate with reduced risk of cardiovascular disease (CVD). After multivariate adjustment an inverse association was observed between consumption of anthocyanidins and coronary heart disease (CHD), CVD, and total mortality and also between flavones and total mortality.[18] A 2006 meta-analysis of 9 cohort studies, comprised of 7 in the U.S.A. and 2 in Finland, considered the risk of CHD in association with the consumption of fruit and vegetable portions. These studies reporting relative risks and quantitative assessments of food intake included 129,701 women, 91,379 men, and 5,007 incidences of CHD events. The risk of CHD decreased significantly by 4% with each additional fruit and vegetable portion daily. The risk reduction was even greater and more significant for fruit alone, with a 7% decrease in risk per portion.[19]

An inverse association was observed between consumption of anthocyanidins and coronary heart disease (CHD), CVD, and total mortality.[18]

Fruit appears beneficial in animal studies through its ability to counteract, reduce, and repair damage due to inflammation and oxidative stress. In addition to flavonoids and phenol acids, other polyphenols in berries that may contribute to their anticancer potential include stilbenoids such as resveratrol and lignans like secoisolariciresinol, as well as nonpolyphenols including triterpenoids such as ursolic acid. Based on *in vitro* studies, complexes of these components in various berry products may also impact enzymes that metabolize carcinogens and help regulate transcription and growth factors and signaling pathways of cancer proliferation, tumor angiogenesis and apoptosis. The sensitization of tumor cells to chemotherapy drugs is another means by which berry fruit may even be of benefit in the treatment of some cancers.[20]

The American Cancer Society website recommendations (as revised on June 30, 2014) are to "eat at least 2½ cups of fruits and vegetables each day" and to "include vegetables and fruits at every meal and snack" to help lower cancer risk. One half-cup serving is 4 ounces.

It is suggested that you "fill half your plate with colorful fruits and vegetables at every meal and eating occasion," but "that *doesn't* mean potato chips!" It also recommends eating "a variety of vegetables and fruits each day." The website also notes that whole fruits and vegetables are to be emphasized, along with choosing 100% juices when drinking fruit beverages, rather than sugar-sweetened fruit-flavored drinks.[21]

The American Heart Association website on healthy diet goals (February 2014) goes even further and suggests at least 4½ cups/day of vegetables and fruit for an average adult, equivalent to 4-5 servings of each per day. [A fruit or vegetable serving is described as 1/2 cup (except a serving for raw leafy vegetables is 1 cup and for dried fruit is 1/4 cup), so at least 9 servings daily of fruits and vegetables are recommended.] It recommends a wide range of vegetables and fruits of different colors (for example a red/green/orange day could include apple/lettuce/carrot) without added salt and sugars. Roasting is a recommended method for cooking vegetables, especially cauliflower, broccoli, Brussels sprouts, onions, carrots, tomatoes or eggplant, to enhance the natural sweetness and reduce bitterness. It also suggests mixing fresh or frozen berries into pancakes, waffles, or muffins, or having fresh, canned (light syrup), or dried fruit or 100% natural fruit juice for dessert.[22]

The bad news is that the trend in America is heading in the wrong direction. The Center for Disease Control nationwide prevalence and trends data shows that, in the 50 United States and 3 American Territories plus the District of Columbia, for 2009 the median percentage of those who consumed fruits and vegetables 5 or more times per day was 23.5%, compared to 24.3% in 2007. In both cases, less than 1 in 4 Americans were consuming at least the minimum recommended intake.[23,24]

> For 2009 the median percentage of those who consumed fruits and vegetables 5 or more times per day was 23.5%, compared to 24.3% in 2007.[23,24]

The Youth Risk Behavior Surveillance report for the U.S.A.

summarized results from a national survey, 39 state surveys, and 22 local surveys of students from grades 9 to 12 during 2007. It showed that only 21.4% of high school students had eaten fruits and vegetables five or more times daily during the 7 days prior to the survey. The percentages declined in going from grade 9 (23.7%) to 10 (22.4%) to 11 (19.9%) to grade 12 (18.6%). In addition, 33.8% had drunk soda pop at least once daily, while only 34.7% achieved the recommended level of physical activity.[25] By 2009 trend for eating fruits and vegetables 5 or more times daily had improved to 22.3% overall, with grade nine (23.0%) still somewhat higher than grade 12 (20.8%), and with daily soda pop consumption (29.2%) and adequate physical activity (37.0%) both showing improvement.[26] However, the results remain poor.

The evidence of flavonoid benefits is found worldwide. For example, in a study published in 2002, the dietary consumption of flavonols and flavonones in foods were examined in 10,054 men and women in Finland and correlated with the risk of developing chronic diseases over a 28-year period. This was based upon dietary recall, the estimated content of flavonoids in Finnish foods, and adjusted for confounding factors including age, sex, locale, occupation, blood pressure, smoking, serum cholesterol, weight, and diabetes. The main sources of 95% of the flavonoids consumed were berries, apples, oranges, grapefruit, juices, onions, and white cabbage. Unfortunately, the consumption of tea and red wine were not assessed, but were considered low; Finns at the time mainly consumed coffee and beer or liquor, respectively, instead. The relative risks between the highest and lowest quartiles (the 25% of the group that consumed the most and the 25% that consumed the least amounts, respectively) of particular flavonoids were compared.[27]

Those in the Finnish study with higher quercetin intake had lower total mortality and lower mortality from ischemic heart disease, lower asthma incidence, lower risk of type 2 diabetes and all cancers, and men had lower lung cancer rates. Men with higher myricetin intake had lower type 2 diabetes and prostate cancer risks. Subjects with higher kaempferol intake had a lower incidence of cerebrovascular disease as well as less thrombosis. Finally, in addition to those flavonols, subjects with higher consumption of flavonones found in citrus fruit, naringenin and hesperetin, also had lower asthma, cerebrovascular disease, and thrombosis incidences. For total flavonol and flavonone consumption, highest consumption was associated with a trend for lower risk for asthma, cerebrovascular disease and thrombosis incidences, and lung cancer risk. Berries, together with apples, were most associated with a lower type 2 diabetes risk. [27]

In a 2012 report on 1898 women of ages 18-75 years from the United Kingdom, data from 1996 to 2007 from food-frequency questionaires was correlated with direct measurements of arterial stiffness and atherosclerosis. Higher anthocyanin intake was associated with significantly lower central systolic blood pressure and pulse wave velocity, an indicater of lower arterial stiffness. The primary sources of anthocyanins in this study were pears (23%), wine (22%), grapes (20%), and berries (13%), especially raspberries and strawberries. Higher flavone intake was also associated with significantly lower pulse wave velocity, as were higher berry and wine intake. It was suggested that 1-2 serving of berries daily is a relevant strategy for reducing cardiovascular risk.[28]

It was suggested that 1-2 serving of berries daily is a relevant strategy for reducing cardiovascular risk.[28]

In a study beginning in Japan in the late 1990s, 77,891 men and women of ages 45-74 years were given a validated food frequency questionnaire to evaluate the association of fruit and vegetable consumption with the risk of total cancer and cardiovascular disease. By the end of 2002 the data showed no association of fruit or vegetable intake with a decreased risk of total cancer, but fruit consumption significantly lowered the risk of cardiovascular disease.[29] While the epidemiological evidence appears compelling, and small-scale randomized controlled trials show improvements in blood pressure, blood lipids, endothelial function, and arterial stiffness with short-term increased consumption of popular berries and anthocyanin extracts, long-term randomized controlled studies need to confirm the benefits of berry polyphenols for cardiovascular health.[30]

⊗Increasing antioxidant consumption lowers the risk of developing some cancers. A review of the worldwide epidemiological literature on the cancer-preventive effects of human consumption of fruits and vegetables found limited evidence for cancers of the mouth, pharynx, esophagus, stomach, colon/recturm, larynx, lung, kidney, bladder (fruit only), and ovary (vegetables only). Based on the range of prevalence of low fruit and vegetable intake, a crude estimate of the percentage of preventable cancers in those with low intake is in the range of 5-12%.[31] ⊗

An integrated series of case-control studies in the 1980s in Italy investigated over 8000 cases of different types of cancer, comparing fruit and vegetable consumption with over 6000 controls admitted to the hospital for noncancerous acute conditions. Using multivariate relative risks to account for normal differences in backgrounds and behaviors, there was a consistent pattern of protection with vegetable consumption for all epithelial cancers (urinary tract, reproductive organs, and the digestive tract and its organs except the gall bladder). For fruit consumption, a strong inverse relationship was found with cancers of the upper digestive and respiratory tracts (mouth, throat, larynx and esophagus) and significant inverse relationships were noted with cancers of the liver, pancreas, prostate, and urinary tract.[32]

For fruit consumption, a strong inverse relationship was found with cancers of the upper digestive and respiratory tracts (mouth, throat, larynx and esophagus) and significant inverse relationships were noted with cancers of the liver, pancreas, prostate, and urinary tract.[32]

When a meta-analysis of 15 case-control studies worldwide and one Japanese cohort study considered the impact of consumption of plant products on oral cancer, it was shown for fruit that each portion consumed per day significantly reduced the risk by 49%, and vegetables similarly reduced the overall risk by 50%.[33]

PROTECTING THE BRAIN AND NERVE FUNCTIONS

The polyphenolics in fruit, vegetables, and beverages (tea, wine, and juices) have also been shown to protect against the processes involved neurodegenerative diseases in animal and based on *in vitro* studies. The mitochondria appears to be the primary target of oxidative damage, especially to the DNA, proteins, and membrane lipids, as the electron transport chain there generate most reactive oxygen species that cause the inflammatory damage. The endogenous free radical scavenging enzymes need supplementation with polyphenolic antioxidants to function most efficiently and slow brain aging and declines in motor and cognitive performance.[34,35]

Neurodegenerative diseases such as Alzheimer's and Parkinson's diseases and amyotrophic lateral sclerosis may potentially be prevented or diminished by substantial dietary intake of polyphenolic compounds such as flavonoids and stilbenes.[34,35] Blueberries in particular have shown preclinical promise in rodents by helping increase hippocampal plasticity, at least in the short term, through multiple mechanims[35,36] including enhanced neuronal signaling that improves motor functions and conversion of short-term to long-term memory.[36] Age-related neurodegenerative diseases are superimposed on behavioral deficits considered a normal aspect of aging. Polyphenolics found in berries provide a nontoxic means of neuroprotection by reducing oxidative stress and inhibiting inflammatory mediators.[37]

The risk of dementia or Alzheimer disease was assessed in 8,085 non-demented subjects over 65 years of age in a 3-city cohort study in France from 1999-2000 and re-examined over 4 years with a follow-up rate of 89%. In fully adjusted models, the daily consumption of fruits and vegetables was associated with a decreased risk of all-cause dementia.[38] Chronic inflammation associated with metabolic syndrome may lead indirectly to dementia from damage to blood vessels. Berry polyphenolics may help reduce cognitive impairment during aging and complicating Alzheimer's disease by their anti-inflammatory protection of vascular function.[39]

> The daily consumption of fruits and vegetables was associated with a decreased risk of all-cause dementia.[38]

Flavonoids, especially the anthocyanins in berries, are potent antioxidant and anti-inflammatory agents that promote anti-aging. Antioxidant capacity alone is not enough to predict the effects against certain aging disorders. A multiplicity of activities such as calcium buffering and cell signalling that differ from one type of berry's phytochemical complex like strawberry compared to another like blueberry, reflected in specific activities in different brain regions, make combinations of berries even more potentially beneficial.[37]

A study prospectively examined the effect of flavonoid consumption from tea, red wine, apples, oranges, and berries on the risk of developing Parkinson disease. It looked at flavonoid consumption for 20-22 years with 80,336 women from the Nurses' Health Study and 49,281 men in the Health Professional Follow-up Study. When comparing the highest and lowest quintiles of flavonoid consumption, after adjusting for multiple confounders in men the hazard risk (HR) was significantly lowered by total flavonoids (HR = 0.60) and the subclasses of berries (HR = 0.77) and anthocyanins (HR = 0.72), but no significant relationships were found for women. This does not exclude the possibility that other constituents in the foods may have also contributed protective effects.[40]

ANTI-INFLAMMATORY BENEFITS OF FRUITS AND VEGETABLES

Low-grade chronic systemic inflammation is associated with a number of chronic disease conditions. Atherosclerosis, one of the main causes of cardiovascular disease, involves T-cells in atherogenic lesions that release pro-inflammatory cytokines and contribute to the growth of plaque. Cancer tumor development, invasion, and metastasis have long been associated with chronic inflammation. Carcinogenesis in particular involves the continual presence of cytokines, chemokines, nuclear factor-kappa B (NF-κB), and reactive oxygen and nitrogen species that can lead to genetic instability and mutations. Obesity is also connected with low-grade inflammation and predisposes individuals to insulin resistance, type 2 diabetes, and metabolic syndrome. Adipose tissue functions as an endocrine organ that secrets pro-inflammatory cytokines like interleukin (IL)-6, tumor necrosis factor-alpha (TNF-α), and other cellular regulators.[41]

Foods that are high in fiber, healthy oils, carotenoids, and flavonoids can help retard these inflammatory changes. Along with whole grains, raw nuts, monounsaturated oils, and omega-3 fatty acids (fish oil), diets high in a variety of vegetables and fruits, especially fruits and berries rich in polyphenols, are associated with lower systemic inflammation. Human studies show the consumption of fruit and vegetables is inversely related to inflammatory marker levels and lowers the risk of cardiovascular disease and metabolic syndrome.[41]

While inflammatory mechanisms are part of normal immune function, when acutely excessive or associated with even low-grade chronic inflammation, tissue damage ensues. Flavonoid polyphenols inhibit pro-inflammatory eicosanoid biosynthesis from arachidonic acids (via cyclooxygenase [COX] and lipoxygenase [LOX]) in part by decreasing neutrophil degranulation (and thereby reducing release of prostaglandins [PG] and leucotrienes [LT], respectively). Plant polyphenols also inhibit inducible nitric oxide synthase (iNOS) expression by macrophages, thus lowering the production of nitric oxide, another crucial inflammation mediator. Polyphenols help reduce prominent pro-inflammatory cytokines such as IL-1, IL-6, and TNF-α by blocking NF-κB and mitogen-activated protein kinase (MAPK) pathways. Suppression of cell adhesion molecule production is another anti-inflammatory mechanism of polyphenols, mediated in part by NF-κB. Finally, polyphenols scavenge reactive oxygen species (ROS) responsible for oxidative stress leading to lipid peroxidation, NF-κB activation, and DNA damage.[41]

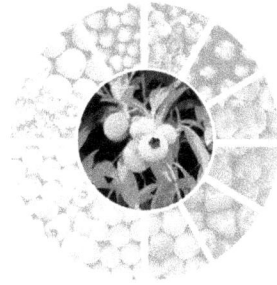

TWO

BERRIES AS NUTRIENT-DENSE FRUIT

BERRIES ARE COMMONLY DESCRIBED AS SMALL, FLESHY FRUIT, LACKING A PIT THAT WOULD BE REMOVED FROM A FRUIT BEFORE EATING, AND MAY CONTAIN MANY SEEDS THAT ARE CONSUMED WITH THE BERRY. THEY ARE USUALLY JUICIER THAN LARGE FRUIT AND LACK A THICK PEEL THAT IS OFTEN REMOVED BEFORE THE CONSUMPTION OF LARGER FRUIT, LEADING TO THE LOSS OF MANY OF THE ANTIOXIDANTS IN THE PEELING PROCESS. BEING SMALLER IN SIZE THAN OTHER FRUIT, BERRIES PROVIDE A HIGHER PROPORTION OF THE COLORED SURFACE THAT IS RICH IN ANTHOCYANINS, IN RELATION TO THE PULP THAT IS GENERALLY MORE PALE AND HIGHER IN SUGARS. CONSEQUENTLY, BERRIES ARE GENERALLY MORE CONCENTRATED IN BENEFICIAL ANTIOXIDANTS AND LOWER IN CALORIES PER UNIT OF WEIGHT THAN LARGER FRUIT.

ANTIOXIDANT ACTIVITY AND PHENOLIC CONTENT OF BERRIES

One of the advantageous effects of consuming berries is the ability of their polyphenolics to prevent cellular oxidative damage. Flavonoids co-exist as complex mixtures in plants with vitamins C and E to act together as hydrogen-donating antioxidants, maintaining the vitamin activities to prevent oxidation in foods, in the GI tract, and systemically. Gallic acid and a majority of flavonoids including anthocyanins have greater antioxidant activity than these two well-known antioxidant vitamins.

They also chelate metals such as iron and copper, thereby preventing free radical generation catalysed by these metalic ions.[1] Each type of polyphenolic compound provides distinctive qualities, while each specific compound within the different polyphenolic categories has its own unique effect.[2]

One possible disadvantage of anthocyanins like cyanidin 3-glucoside, compared to flavonols like quercetin, may be their less complete absorption,[3] though this perceived difference may be due to anthocyanin conversion and/or their incomplete measurement if protein-bound in the blood.[4] The benefits of consuming whole berries derive from the complexity of the nutrient content, and this can be vastly expanded by using different kinds of berries together, especially those from different taxonomic genera, thereby expanding the phenolic variability and activities.[4]

> The benefits of consuming whole berries derive from the complexity of the nutrient content, and this can be vastly expanded by using different kinds of berries together, especially those from different taxonomic genera, thereby expanding the phenolic variability and activities.[4]

For example, two anthocyanins (cyanidin-3-rutinoside and cyanidin-3-glucosylrutinoside) in red raspberries (*R. idaeus*) are especially potent antioxidants, comparable to the preservatives BHA and BHT and superior to vitamin E at 125 mcg/ml. These anthocyanins are also potent inhibitors of COX-1 and especially COX-2, comparable to the anti-inflammatory drugs ibuprofen and naproxen at 10 mcM concentrations. Black raspberries (*R. occidentalis*) also contain one of these anthocyanins (cyanidin-3-rutinoside), but cranberries and blueberries (*Vaccinium* spp.) contain neither. Anthocyanins from raspberries and blackberries (*Rubus* spp.) at 125 mcg/ml are also potent antioxidants and inhibitors of COX-1 (45.8% and 38.5%, respectively) and COX-2 (31.2% and 45.7%, respectively), while those in cranberries and blueberries at the same concentration are much less active inhibitors of COX-1 (15.5% and 9.1%, respectively) and COX-2 (14.7% and 10.1%, respectively).[5]

The absolute amount by percentage of dry weight of all antioxidant components (including polyphenols, carotenoids, glutathione, and vitamins C and E) in items in the American diet is greatest for culinary herbs and spices. However, based on typical serving sizes, in order of rank the five richest sources of these compounds are blackberries, walnuts, strawberries, artichokes, and cranberries, while raspberries and blueberries are also included in the top ten.[6] A preferred means of measuring antioxidant activity is the oxygen radical absorbance capacity (ORAC) that can be applied both to protection of either fat-based (lipophilic) or water-based (hydrophilic) substances. The hydrophilic ORAC values for most plant foods is much greater than for lipophilic antioxidant activity. The fresh fruit with the highest hydrophilic ORAC per serving are the blueberry, cranberry, blackberry, strawberry, and raspberry.[7]

The antioxidant score determined by total oxyradical scavenging capacity indicates that cranberry is highest. When measuring the total phenolic content in fruit and including both freely soluble and bound forms, the highest amount is also found in cranberry.[8] The total phenolic content is generally greater in berries than in other fresh fruit, and, even then, the highest ratio of hydrophilic ORAC to total phenolics in fresh fruit is found with cranberry, blueberry, apple, peach, sweet cherry, apricot, strawberry, raspberry, and blackberry, in that order.[7]

AMERICAN BERRIES AS TRADITIONAL FOOD AND REMEDIES

It does not require great insight to perceive that the native berries in America served as an important food source for the indigenous people and the early colonists and pioneers who settled in the regions where various species grew naturally. It is documented that cranberries and lowbush and highbush blueberries (*Vaccinium* spp.) were eaten raw or cooked, dried for winter or as a trail food while hunting, and/or were mixed in cornbread and pemmican by the natives in what is now northeastern America and southeastern Canada. Black raspberries and blackberries (*Rubus* spp.) were used similarly in a broader distribution, while chokeberry (*Aronia melanocarpa*) consumption appeared more localized and limited to use of fresh berries.[9] It is not surprising that many of these berries were selectively cultivated, based on the most desirable properties for production including features involved in optimizing growth, handling, harvested, and preserving.

There is little evidence that early Euro-American settlers recognized or utilized the fruit of American native wild berries for major health purposes other than as foods. Blackberries (*Rubus villosus*) were considered remedies for diarrhea when eaten in large quantities, but this effect was more prominent with the root of the plant which came to be preferred for that use. The berries or juice were added to other remedies to improve the flavor, so that the well-known blackberry cordial was prepared by boiling down berries in water, along with spices such as cinnamon, cloves, and allspice, and the adding sugar and whiskey to preserve it. This type of preparation was considered a standard remedy for diarrhea.[10,11]

This blackberry cordial folk remedy was further elaborated by Dr. Cook in the Physiomedical Dispensatory in 1869 and described as having many formulas, but he noted that the berries alone were often the only corrector needed. The only "*Vaccinium* species" berries described by Cook were huckleberries (*Gaylussacia resinosa*, formerly *Vaccinium resinosum*) and whortleberries (*G. frondosa*, formerly *V. frondosum*) who described these, "and probably of other species of the *Vaccinium*," as acting on the kidneys as mild diuretics in cases of dropsy.[12] At the end of the 19th century, *King's American Dispensatory* quoted the *United States Pharmacopeia* in mentioning the fruit of black raspberrry and American red raspberry (*R. strigosus*) as being employed in place of red raspberry (*R. idaeus*) fruit for making a flavoring syrup or diluted for use as a pleasant drink in fevers. The blackberry syrup was used similarly, and blackberry syrup, jam and jelly were added to water for treating diarrhea or dysentery. Under the description of whortleberries ("*Vaccinium*"), the fruit of the "related species" cranberry was described as being applied in domestic practice as a poultice for inflammatory swellings such as erysipelas and indolent ulcers, or as "recently recommended by a distinguished physician," split and applied with a daub of flour paste over a boil on the tip of the nose.[13]

By the mid-20th century, the *Naturopathic Dispensatory* described only the rootbark of blackberry and red raspberry as being used for treating diarrhea, while no mention of cranberry is made.[14] Along with the roots, the leaves of blackberry and red raspberry were also described in Dr. John Lust's *The Herb Book* for their astringency in controlling diarrhea, while American red raspberry fruit were described as mildly laxative and the berry juice as a refrigerant beverage for fevers. Fresh berry juices in general were advocated to enhance general well being.[15] Though flavonoid glycosides in general were considered as "vitamin P", acting as synergists with vitamin C for preserving the integrity of vascular walls, the anthocyanin pigments in fruits and berries were not specifically mentioned in the *Naturopathic Dispensatory* in this context.[14]

The protective powers of these and other related components in berries were appreciated in general, if not for the specific health purposes that were recognized in the latter half of the century. The usefulness of native berries in regard to preventing disease attracted popular attention when application in the Cape Cod area of the juice of the cranberry as a means of addressing urinary tract infections was first investigated in 1959[16] and further examined during the following decades.

❖ An examination of recent research on a few of the most popular native American berries reveals that much is being learned about the value of their consumption not only as food but for helping prevent development of some of the most debilitating and deadly chronic diseases that have become epidemic in America and constitute a growing worldwide pandemic. The impact of these simple dietary items on risk factors for neurodegenerative and cardiovascular disease and cancer has much to do with the berries' antioxidant and anti-inflammatory influences. ❖

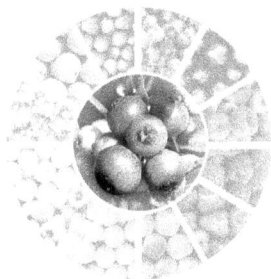

THREE

HEATH FAMILY *VACCINIUM* BERRIES

PLANTS OF THE FAMILY ERICACEAE (HEATH OR HEATHER) THAT ARE IN THE
VACCINIUM GENUS PROVIDE SOME OF THE MOST POPULAR BERRIES IN
NORTH AMERICA AND EUROPE. THERE ARE MANY DIFFERENT CULTIVARS
OR VARIETIES OF COMMERCIAL VACCINIUM SPECIES, FOR ADAPTATION TO
DIFFERENT SOILS AND CLIMATES. ALONG WITH AMERICAN CRANBERRY
V. MACROCARPON, THE LOWBUSH V. ANGUSTIFOLIUM, HIGHBUSH
V. CORYMBOSUM, AND RABBITEYE V. ASHEI BLUEBERRY SPECIES WILL
BE FEATURED HERE AS IMPORTANT FOODS FOR PROTECTING AND
MAINTAINING HEALTH AND AVOIDING CHRONIC DISEASES.

Major blueberry species thrive in the colder north where the
required number of chilling hours to bear fruit are easily met. In fact,
blueberries are Canada's largest fruit crop. The wild lowbush blueberry
(*V. angustifolium*) dominates some landscapes to the extent that they are
harvested commercially by certain indigenous American and Canadian
peoples. However, the most common commercial blueberry species
remains the cultivated northern highbush blueberry (*V. corymbosum*).
Though native to eastern Canada and in the United States as far west
as Wisconsin and south to Alabama, highbush blueberry varieties have
also been introduced commercially into the Pacific regions of both
countries.

In the South, the rabbiteye blueberry (*V. ashei* syn. *V. virgatum*) received its name from the appearance of the pinkish-white unripe berries that resemble the eyes of an albino rabbit. It is joined in the southeast from Virginia to Florida to Texas by the Elliott's blueberry or Mayberry (*V. elliotti*) [not to be confused with the Elliot cultivar of *V. corymbosum*] that has a late-season, somewhat more sour berry, leading to rabbiteye blueberry being more commecially popular. The rabbiteye blueberry becomes available earlier in the year before northern highbush varieties, but recent southern highbush hybrids of rabbiteye blueberry or the Darrow's evergreen blueberry (*V. darrowi*) with *V. corymbosum* has resulted in low-chill varieties of superior quality fruit available earlier than rabbiteye. Utilizing these developments in southern Florida and California and along their coasts, it has now become possible to commercially cultivate more blueberries in warmer climates.

Of the three species of cranberry, only the *V. macrocarpon*, sometimes called American cranberry, originated exclusively on the North American continent. Two other species also grow in the northern regions of this continent, the bog cranberry (*V. oxycoccus*) and the small cranberry (*V. microcarpum*), but their natural range also extends into northern Europe and northern Asia. Since American cranberry is the primary commercial cranberry because of its larger size, most study has been done on this species, so it will be considered here. Native to the Northeast, cranberries are also grown commercially in Wisconsin and the Pacific Northwest and the Canadian provinces adjacent to all of these states.

Other European *Vaccinium* species that are cultivated include the red lingonberry (*V. vitis-idaea*) and dark blue bilberry (*V. myrtillus*). In America, their wild counterparts may be considered the red huckleberry (*V. parvilorum*) and the black mountain huckleberry (*V. membranaceum*). However, the most popular of the North American *Vaccinium* berries are the commercial species of blueberries.

Research data on different cranberry and blueberry cultivars will be combined for each species. Studies on the different blueberry species will identify each, when characterized in the research, to help distinguish potential differences between these species. When unspecified, the research may be generically applicable to blueberries. Due to the great diversity of cultivars for cultivated species, these are not specified.

Blueberries

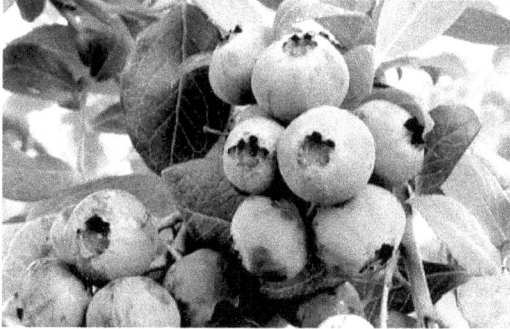

LOWBUSH, HIGHBUSH, AND RABBITEYE

BLUEBERRIES ARE ONE OF THE MOST POPULAR BERRIES IN AMERICA TODAY, WITH SEVERAL MAJOR COMMERCIAL SPECIES. EVEN THOUGH A VARIETY OF CULTIVARS AND HYBRIDS OF BLUEBERRY SPECIES HAVE BEEN DEVELOPED TO HELP MAXIMIZE AGRICULTURAL PRODUCTION, COMMON COMPONENTS GIVE THESE BERRIES THE COLOR AND FLAVOR CHARACTERISTICS SO WELL KNOWN AND ENJOYED AND THE BIOACTIVITY DESIRABLE FOR BETTER HEALTH. THE TYPES OF ANTHOCYANINS AND METABOLITES THAT TYPIFY THESE BERRIES EFFECTIVELY PENETRATE INTO BRAIN TISSUE, UNLIKE OTHER COMPOUNDS BLOCKED BY THE "BLOOD-BRAIN BARRIER". THIS ALLOWS THESE COMPONENTS TO HELP PROTECT FUNCTIONAL MEMORY. IN ADDITION, BLUEBERRY POLYPHENOLS IMPROVE OVERALL OXIDATIVE STATUS AND CARDIOVASCULAR HEALTH, WHILE HELPING MAINTAIN NORMAL BLOOD SUGAR LEVELS.

The wild, or lowbush, blueberries are grown in eastern Canada and northeastern United States. Lowbush blueberry leaf color and plant size are variable in the wild, whereas cultivars in highbush plantations produce fields and berries that are uniform in appearance. Highbush blueberries, distinguished by the plant size in comparison to the lowbush species, are cultivated in temperate areas of the USA, especially the Great Lakes region, the Pacific Northwest, and in the Atlantic states. Lowbush and highbush blueberries produce similar harvest levels in North America, and together provide between 170-193 million kg annually. Though fresh blueberries are almost always highbush varieties, some highbush blueberries are frozen. Lowbush blueberries are first frozen and then mainly used in processed foods such as muffins, pastry fillings, jams, and sauces.[1]

In the South, rabbiteye blueberries (*V. ashei* syn. *V. virgatum*), native to southern Georgia, southeast Alabama, and the Florida panhandle, are now grown commercially from Virginia to Texas, as they are generally more productive in this region than the northern species. They grow taller (over 10 ft.) than the highbush blueberries, and the berries ripen over a several week period. Rabbiteye berries are smaller and have a thicker skin than the highbush berries. They are somewhat sweeter when eaten fresh, but can have a grittiness due to seeds and stone cells. While rabbiteye berries have a longer shelf-life than highbush berries, they are typically used in syrups, sauces, or baking. Rabbiteye blueberries are more resistant to pests and disease, but they require cross-pollination by bees, usually blueberry bees and bumblebees.

POLYPHENOLIC COMPONENT COMPARISONS BETWEEN BLUEBERRY SPECIES AND WITH CRANBERRIES

The lowbush blueberries, 80% of which are between 0.15-0.3 g/berry, are more uniform in size than the highbush blueberries, 60% of which are 0.5-1.5 g/berry, but 30% 1.5-2.5, g/berry. Both lowbush and highbush blueberry pigment is found only in the skin of the fruit. Though much smaller in size, wild lowbush blueberries are by fresh weight on average significantly higher in total phenolics, anthocyanins, and oxygen radical absorbance capacity (ORAC) antioxidant activity than cultivated highbush varieties. The lowbush berries contained almost two times more total phenolics than the highbush berries by fresh weight. The variations in anthocyanins and total phenolics within species were similar for both lowbush and highbush blueberries, less than 2-fold differences in the 10th and 90th percentiles for each species. These phenolics are negatively affected by processing treatments that expose the berries to heat and air.[1]

In contrast, a study of all 3 species found the total phenolic content, anthocyanins, and ORAC on average to be similar among them but also to vary widely among a half dozen different cultivars for the northern highbush blueberry and 4 cultivars of rabbiteye blueberry. Great increases in these parameters were seen in 2 cultivars from Georgia when rabbiteye blueberry was harvested very late (July 28), compare to normal harvest time. On the other hand, the phytochemical contents and ORACs were mostly similar in the same highbush cultivar (Jersey) grown variously in New Jersey, Michigan, and Oregon. The ORAC was related linearly to both the anthocyanin and total phenolic contents. Only a single lowbush blueberry sample was tested.[2]

A study of all 3 species found the total phenolic content, anthocyanins, and ORAC on average to be similar among them.[2]

Comparing freeze-dried powders of highbush and lowbush blueberries revealed the lowbush berries yield the highest chlorogenic acid amounts. Organically grown highbush blueberries had higher flavanol oligimers and chlorogenic acid than those conventionally grown, but lower anthocyanin content. Phenolic content levels varied between cultivars, with broad ranges for the main anthocyanidins of both species: delphinidin, malvidin, and petunidin ranging from 45-75 mg, 34-63 mg, and 21-36 mg per 100 grams fresh weight, respectively.[3]

Blueberrry resveratrol content varies by cultivar and region.[4] Highbush blueberries from Michigan showed good resveratrol content but the highbush berries from British Columbia completely lacked resveratrol. Lowbush blueberries from Nova Scotia were intermediate.[5] Highbush blueberry from Oregon also contains the stilbene piceatannol (186-422 ng/g), and rabbiteye blueberries from Mississippi yield pterostilbene (99-151 ng/g).[4] Pterostilbene, like resveratrol, is a potent antioxidant and chemopreventive agent.[6]

Lowbush blueberries even have almost 75% greater total phenolic content than cranberries.[7] Being of the same genus as cranberries, blueberries have some phytochemicals and attributes in common with their red cousins. Highbush blueberries contains the flavonoids quercetin and myricetin, though cranberries are significantly higher in these flavonols than blueberries.[8] Lowbush blueberries and cranberries collected in the wild in Nova Scotia contain substantial resveratrol (863 and 900 ng/g dried, respectively), while highbush and rabbiteye cultivars grown in the United States show great variation (327-1074 and 7-1691 ng/g dried, respectively).[4]

As is easily perceived by the colors, the anthocyanins of blueberries and cranberries are distinctive. Highbush blueberries contains predominantly malvidin, delphinidin, and petunidin 3-glycosides and smaller amounts of cyanidin and peonidin 3-glucosides,[3,9-12] rabbiteye cultivars have mostly malvidin, peonidin, and cyanidin and less petunidin and delphinidin,[13] whereas the main anthocyanins of cranberry are mainly peonidin 3-glycosides and less cyandin 3-glycosides.[10,14]

The anthocyanin and phenolic acid contents of 6 commercial blueberry cultivars and 4 breeding selections were tested in frozen berries and ranged between 201.4 - 402.8 mg/100g and 23.6 - 61.7 mg/100g, respectively. The main anthocyanins on average were 3-0-arabinosides and 3-0-galactosides of delphinidin, cyanidin, and malvidin, while the phenolic acids measured were over 96% chlorogenic acid. The 3 genotypes that contained highest amounts of the 3-0-glucosides of malvidin, delphinidin, and cyanidin are the cultivar O'Neal and breeding selections NC4900 and SHF2B-1 21:3. These 3 also had the highest total phenolic acid/chlorogenic acid contents of the 10 tested. Malvidin-3-0-glucoside and chlorogenic acid are major hypoglycemic principles.[15]

BLUEBERRY ANTIOXIDANT ACTIVITY

IN HUMANS

After 14 healthy subjects were fed a high-carbohydrate and low-fat breakfast (1 cup of cornflakes with 1/2 cup of 2% milk) together with 12.5 or 5.8 grams of freeze-dried blueberry powder (obtained from 75 grams [1/2 cup serving] or 35 grams of fresh blueberries, respectively) or a placebo control with equivalent vitamin C and sugars as the high berry dose, the serum ORAC was measured for the following 3 hours and compared to fasting values. Each person received all 3 treatments with a week in between, and the average effects for each treatment showed that the high berry dose produced a significantly higher ORAC than placebo after 1 and 2 hours and a significantly higher ORAC than the low berry dose after 2 hours. This demonstrates that the increased antioxidant capacity from blueberries in humans is not due simply to the vitamin C and fructose content.[16]

In a randomized, placebo-controlled, crossover study 18 male healthy male subjects of average age 47.8 years, 25 g of wild lowbush blueberry freeze-dried powder, equivalent to 1 cup (148 g) of raw blueberries and providing 375 mg of anthocyanins, and placebo were each given as a drink for 6 weeks, with a 6-week washout in between the 2 treatments. The wild blueberry drink led to significant reductions in levels of endogenously oxidized DNA bases and hydrogen peroxide-induced DNA damage, whereas the placebo drink produced no effect.[17]

> The wild blueberry drink led to significant reductions in levels of endogenously oxidized DNA bases and hydrogen peroxide-induced DNA damage, whereas the placebo drink produced no effect.[17]

IN ANIMALS

In mice fed 600 mg blueberries per 10 grams of body weight for 21 days, liver antioxidant markers were significantly increased compared to controls, while the liver oxidative marker was lower, showing liver protection from oxidative stress. The blueberry group also had significantly increased proliferation of splenic lymphocytes, especially the CD3+ and the CD4+ T lymphocyte subsets.[18] A 70% aqueous acetone extract of wild lowbush blueberries at 50 mcg/ml was able to inhibit the *in vitro* oxidation of the hydrophilic amino acid tyrosine and the lipophilic fatty acid linoleic acid. Free radicals were quenched most effectively *in vitro* by the two fractions that were highest in flavanols, anthocyanins, and phenolic acids.[19] The *in vivo* and *in vitro* laboratory results support the human findings that blueberries provide antioxidant protection.

ANTIOXIDANT COMPARISONS WITH OTHER BERRIES AND FRUITS

To determine whether a meal of different types and/or forms of berries or fruits cause significant changes in plasma antioxidant capacity as measured by ORAC, 5 clinical trials each with 6-10 human subjects used a crossover design to compare relatively equivalent amounts of wild blueberry and dried plum, Bing sweet cherry, and strawberry, kiwifruit, and red grape. The fresh wild blueberry and cherry increased the lipophilic antioxidant capacity, while fresh and freeze-dried wild blueberries and freeze-dried grape increased hydrophilic antioxidant capacity.[20]

A recently developed assay for measuring cellular antioxidant activity (CAA) that accounts for aspects of uptake, metabolism and location of antioxidants in cells shows that wild blueberry had greater activity than cranberry, apple, and red or green grapes. The most potent compound tested for CAA was quercetin, then kaempferol, epigallocatechin gallate, myricetin, and luteolin, in that order.[7] Highbush blueberries also contain substantial quercetin glycosides, and altogether its polyphenolics and vitamin C provide much greater total antioxidant activity than European cranberries (*V. oxycoccus*), based on FRAP assays.[12]

Phenolic compounds vary between *Vaccinium* species. Highbush blueberries are very high in chlorogenic acid, and contain as much quercetin glycosides as lingonberry (*V. vitis-idaea*) and more than American cranberry.[10] From a molecular perspective, the antioxidant capacity of anthocyanins increases with hydroxyl substitutions on the B-ring, whereas the substitution of methoxyl groups reduces the antioxidant activity. Anthocyanins with a hydroxyl substitution at position 3 on ring C demonstrate a potent antioxidant activity.[21]

Compared to strawberries and blackberries, rabbiteye blueberries showed greater total antioxidant capacity (according to ABTS and DPPH method) and total phenolic, total flavonoid, and total anthocyanin contents.[22] When rabbiteye blueberries were compared to bilberries (*V. myrtillus*), black currant (*Ribes nigrum*), chokeberry (*Aronia melanocarpa*), and elderberry (*Sambucus nigra*), the 15 anthocyanins of the 2 *Vaccinium* species were identical, though distribution patterns differed. Chokeberry (4), elderberry (4), and black currant (6) had fewer anthocyanins. Antioxidant activities by the DPPH method were similar, but they diminished in order from bilberry to rabbiteye blueberry, black currant, chokeberry, and then elderberry.[23]

BLUEBERRY COMPONENTS COUNTER INFLAMMATION TO LOWER CHRONIC DISEASE RISK

Chronic inflammation is a major contributing factor for many progressive disease conditions, including cardiovascular disease, neurological disorders, obesity, metabolic disorders, connective tissue diseases, chronic inflammatory diseases, and cancer. Blueberries are a major sources of anthocyanidins such as cyanidin and delphinidin, along with proanthocyanidins, that help reduce inflammatory risks including oxidative damage.[24]

IN ANIMALS

Obese and lean rats were fed a control diet or one enriched with 8% freeze-dried wild lowbush blueberries, containing 1.5% of 21 different anthocyanins (mainly malvidin- and peonidin-3-galactoside), for 8 weeks and monitored for pro-inflammatory status associated with metabolic syndrome. The obese rats fed blueberries showed significant reductions in plasma TNF-α, IL-6, and C-reactive protein (CRP), and increased adiponectin compared to controls. Expression of CRP in the liver was also significantly down-regulated by blueberries by -25% and for TNF-α, IL-6, and NF-κB in the liver by -59%, -65%, and -25%, respectively, with significant reductions also in abdominal fat tissue. Similar trends were seen for the lean mice given blueberries, with significant liver reductions in TNF-α and NF-κB of -50% and -24%, respectively, and increased adiponectin of +25%. The results indicate a greater overall effect in reducing inflammatory markers in the obese rat, a model of metabolic syndrome.[26]

IN VITRO

Of anthocyanins at 40 mcM concentrations, cyanidin and malvidin had the greatest inhibition on cyclooxygenase (COX)-1 (52% and 48%, respectively) and COX-2 (74% and 65%, respectively) and contribute to the anti-inflammatory effects.[25]

BIOAVAILABILITY OF BLUEBERRY ANTHOCYANINS

IN HUMANS

When 189 grams of lowbush blueberries with 690 mg total anthocyanins were fed to 6 elderly women, urine samples contained 22 of the 24 anthocyanins in amounts that reasonably correlated with the presence in the berries. Though no plasma levels were detected, methylation of cyanidin to peonidin and glucuronide conjugate formation were demonstrated. Overall, absorption of anthocyanins was low in comparison to other flavonoids, as shown in this and other studies, based on plasma levels and urine recovery.[27] On the other hand, after 5 middle-aged men were fed 100 grams of freeze-dried lowbush blueberry powder with 1.2 grams of 25 different anthocyanins (42% of the total phenolics), 19 were detected in the serum. The anthocyanin presence in the serum was correlated with a significantly increased antioxidant capacity *ex vivo*.[28]

IN ANIMALS

Highbush blueberry anthocyanins were not detected in the plasma or urine after being fed to fasting pigs, but they were identified in all four tissues examined including the liver, eye, cortex and cerebellum, indicating that they passed intact beyond the blood-brain barrier. Malvidin in particular was most apparent in all tissues, and though galactosides predominated in the liver, the glucosides were showed more absorption in the brain.[29] When blueberries were fed to pigs at 2.4-12 mg/kg body weight of anthocyanin daily for 4 weeks, the concentration in the whole eye was 0.709 ng/g. Since the pigs were fasted for 18 hours before tissue collection, when no anthocyanins were present in the plasma, they must have collected in the tissue. When comparing diets for pigs with 0%, 1%, 2%, or 4% of the diet as blueberries, the amount of accumulation correlated with increased intake.[30]

When pigs were fed freeze-dried highbush blueberries as 2% of the diet for 8 weeks, the anthocyanins were found in the brain with similar concentrations in the cortex, cerebellum, and midbrain and diencephalon. Fewer types of anthocyanins were in the cortex, though malvidin-3-glucoside was the most abundant in all regions, probably due to its metabolic generation locally as a metabolite along with its passing the blood-brain barrier. Similarly, peonidin-3-glucoside was relatively abundant in all areas in proportionally higher concentrations in the brain than in the blueberries themselves, likely to its generation via methylation of cyanidin-3-glucoside.[31]

In 19-month-old rats fed a 2% blueberry water extract diet for 8-10 weeks, anthocyanins containing malvidin, delphinidin, peonidin, and cyanidin were fround in the cortex, hippocampus, cerebellum, and striatum. (No petunidin glycosides were found in the berries or extract.) The total number of these compounds present in the cortex correlated with improved performance in a water maze, suggesting their central signal modifying capabilities.[32]

INTESTINAL INFLUENCES OF BLUEBERRIES

IN HUMANS

When 25 grams of freeze-dried wild lowbush blueberries were consumed in 250 ml of water daily for 6 weeks by 20 healthy males with an average age of 46 years, relative content of *Bifidobacteria* spp. was significantly increased. *Lactobacillus* spp. also increased, but this likewise occurred after 6 weeks of a placebo drink, whereas there were no significant changes in other intestinal flora. Both *Bifidobacteria* and *Lactobacillus* are considered to be a beneficial factors for digestion and in gut and immune health and are typically included in many probiotic products. Therefore, wild blueberries can be considered as a potential prebiotic functional food, likely due to their anthocyanin, vitamin K, and fiber content.[33]

In Vitro

The impact of metabolism on rabbiteye blueberry phenolic acids by microbes from the colon of different human volunteers influences the inflammatory pathways in colon cells in different ways, resulting in variable effects dependent on the intestinal flora.[34]

Influences on Cognitive Function

In Humans

An extraordinary follow-up evaulation in the Nurses' Health study began from 1995-2001 to measure cognitive function in 16,010 women that were over the age of 70 years to assess whether dietary patterns may have an influence on memory. After adjusting for multiple potential confounders, the cognitive decline differences were determined for dietary intake of particular foods. It was discovered that greater intakes of total flavonoids in general and anthocyanins in particular were associated with slower rates of declining memory. Consuming blueberries once or more per week, compared to less than once per month, was associated with a significant reduction in the average rate of global cognitive decline. The only other comparable food in this study was strawberries, for which consumption twice or more weekly versus less than once weekly reduced the mean decline in global score. These results suggest a delay of cognitive aging of 1.5-2.5 years for those who eat blueberries or strawberries once or twice per week, respectively.[35]

> Consuming blueberries once or more per week, compared to less than once per month, was associated with a significant reduction in the average rate of global cognitive decline. [35]

The protection and preservation of mental capabilities cannot be over-rated, especially as one ages. The tendency for a decline in memory and other cognitive functions in the elderly can be addressed even before it is detected. A study with 9 older adults with an average age of 76.2 years examined the effect of lowbush blueberry juice supplementation on memory. The dose varied by body weight (6-9 mg/kg), ranging from

444 ml to 621 ml daily for 12 weeks. At the end of the study period, word list recall and paired associated learning were significantly improved. Compared with a demographically matched sample of 7 adults using a placebo beverage in a companion trial, paired associate learning were again significantly improved.[36]

In Animals

Most work in the area of memory protection has been done in Alzheimer disease models in rats. Feeding freeze-dried water extract of fresh blueberries as 2% of the diet from 4 until 12 months of age to rats with transgenic predisposition to developing amyloid beta alterations resulted in enhancement of neuronal signaling associated with memory and beneficially altered phospholipase C activity compared to controls. This indicate that overcoming the genetic predisposition to Alzheimer's disease may be possible.[37] The same fresh blueberry extract was homogenized in water and centrifuged to remove the fiber and then freeze-dried. When given as 2% of the diet fed to 4-month-old rats for 2 weeks, it improved cognitive performance in a water maze compared to controls, even more than the NSAID drug piroxicam, by reducing inflammatory expression induced by the neurotoxic kainic acid injection in the hippocampus. The extract group alone augmented expression of the neurotropic factor insulin-like growth factor-1 (IGF-1).[38]

Again, this same preparation (homogenizing fresh blueberries in water, centrifuging the homogenate, and freeze-drying the liquid supernatant), providing on average 394 mg per day of freeze-dried blueberry extract, derived from about 4.4 g/day of fresh blueberries, resulted in aged rats performing similarly in visual object recognition memory tasks as young rats and significantly better than aged controls. The nuclear factor kappa-B (NF-κB) pro-inflammatory transcription factor levels of the aged rats fed blueberry water extract were significantly lower than in the aged controls in 4 of 5 brains regions, and this correlated with memory scores.[39] When a 2% rabbiteye blueberry water extract diet was fed to aged rats for 2 months, the object memory at 19 months was significantly better than for controls, and the improvement was retained a month after stopping blueberries. In 20-month-old rats, object memory scores improved with 2% blueberry diet for 1 month, while for controls it declined; the differences were significant.[40]

Memory decline in aging is associated with reduced new growth of neurons in the hippocampus. Factors associated with learning and memory, like IGF-1 and its activation of extracellular receptor kinase (ERK) and new nerve growth, are all significantly increased and correlate with improved spatial memory in aged rats also supplemented with the 2% blueberry freeze-dried extract diet for 8 weeks, compared to controls.[41]

Also, after 8 weeks of blueberry water extract supplementation in 19-month-old rats, motor behavioral performance was improved for several tasks, along with reversals in biochemical aging parameters for neuronal activities.[42] Rabbiteye blueberry and cranberry extracts were superior to blackcurrant and boysenberry (*Rubus loganbaccus*) fruit extracts, when supplied as 2% of the diet of aged 19-month old rats, for ameliorating motor functional deficits and providing hippocampal neuroprotection. The polyphenols in these 2 *Vaccinium* species also improved muscle tone, strength and balance, as well as enhancing neuronal functioning and response to stress.[43]

Rats fed a diet with 14.3% fresh lowbush blueberries for 6 weeks received carotid artery ligation to simulate a stroke and were compared to others that were ligated but received no blueberries. A 40% loss of neurons in the hippocampus of the associated cerebral hemisphere in the controls was reduced to a 17% loss in those receiving blueberries, indicating a potential for improving ischemic stroke outcomes.[44]

Anti-aging effects of blueberries may be due in part to stilbene components. Pterostilbene at 0.004% of the diet (40 mg/kg in the feed) in 19-month-old rats was effective in improving working memory compared to controls, and at 0.016% of the diet further reduced the effects of aging on cognitive performance that correlated with measurable pterostilbene in the hippocampal tissue. Both doses protected against decreased dopamine release after exposure to oxidative stress to striatal tissue *ex vivo*.[45] Rabbiteye blueberries that contain pterostilbene[31] significantly increased the survival of embryonic dopamine neurons transplanted into dopamine-depleted striatum when the freeze-dried water extract was given as 2% of the diet to rats. This could theoretically improve dopamine neuron transplantation in Parkinson disease patients.[46]

In Vitro

Effects of lowbush blueberry acetic-methanolic extract rich in polyphenolics included protection against hydrogen peroxide-induced oxidative damage and cell death in human neuronal cells, while amyloid-beta aggregation was inhibited at 15 mcg/ml. Pro-oxidant effects were seen in embryonic kidney cells.[47] The 12% water and 88% methanol solvent has been shown to be best for extracting the total phenolics and highest anthocyanin contents and antioxidant capacity.[1]

Impact on Metabolic Syndrome

Metabolic syndrome is a constellation of conditions commonly associated in the modern world. It is characterized by abdominal obesity, impaired glucose tolerance, high triglycerides and low HDL cholesterol, high blood pressure, oxidative stress and inflammation, and an increased risk of type 2 diabetes and atherosclerotic cardiovascular disease. Insulin resistance plays a key role. As such, blueberries and cranberries both offer a number of benefits in helping to prevent or ameliorate this condition.[48]

In Humans

In looking at food intake questionnaires of 46,672 and 87,242 women in Nurses Health Study (NHS) I & II, respectively, and 23,043 men in Health Professions Follow-Up Study (HPFUS) who were without heart disease, high blood pressure or treatment for hypertension, a 14-year follow-up found 5629 cases of hypertension in men and 29,018 cases in women. They found those of age 60 years or over who consumed blueberries more than once per week had a 10% reduction in hypertension risk compared to no blueberry intake. The top quintile (20%) overall of anthocyanin users had a significant 8% reduced risk of high blood pressure, compared to the lowest 20% of anthocyanin consumers. The risk reduction for those 60 years of age or older, when comparing the highest and lowest quintiles, was significant for cyanidin, malvidin, peonidin, and petunidin anthocyanins.[49]

Those of age 60 years or over who consumed blueberries more than once per week had a 10% reduction in hypertension risk compared to no blueberry intake. [49]

In pooling the data from NHS I (70,359; 1984-2008) and II (89,201; 1991-2007) and HPFUS (41,334; 1986-2006) to evaluate diet influence on the development of type 2 diabetes, blueberry consumption twice or more per week significantly reduced the risk of diabetes compared to those who ate blueberries less than once per month.[50] A more recent examination of the pooled data from the NHS I (66,105; 1984-2008) and II (1991-2009) and HPFUS (36,173; 1986-2008) confirmed that for type 2 diabetes the hazard ratio of 0.74 for every 3 servings of blueberries per week was the lowest of all fruit. This is well ahead of the pooled hazard ratios for 3 servings/week of 0.88 for grapes/raisins, 0.89 for prunes, and 0.93 for apples/pears, while the hazard ratio of 1.08 for consumption of fruit juice indicates its association with a higher risk of type 2 diabetes.[51]

Blueberry consumption twice or more per week significantly reduced the risk of diabetes compared to those who ate blueberries less than once per month.[50]

To examine the effect of blueberries on insulin sensitivity, a randomized, double-blind, placebo-controlled trial studied 15 obese, insulin-resistant men and women who utilized 22.5 grams of freeze-dried blueberry combination (1:1 highbush and rabbiteye) in a smoothie, versus 17 who had none in their smoothie, twice daily for 6 weeks. Insulin sensitivity improved significantly more in the blueberry group, though percent body fat, energy intake, serum glucose, lipid profile, blood pressure, and inflammatory biomarkers did not change significantly.[52]

In a single-blind, randomized, controlled 8-week study with 44 women and 4 men averaging 50 years of age and obese with metabolic syndrome, 25 grams of freeze-dried blueberries (1:1 highbush and rabbiteye) in 480 ml of water was consumed twice daily by 25 subjects, and an equivalent amount of water only was taken by the 23 controls. The daily freeze-dried blueberries taken by 25 subjects was equivalent to 350 g of fresh berries. While the systolic and diastolic blood pressure reductions were significantly greater in the berry group than in controls, there were no changes in serum glucose or lipid profiles. However, those using the berries had significantly greater reductions in lipid peroxidation markers, including oxidized LDL.[53]

Since postmenopausal women often develop arterial stiffness and high blood pressure, an 8-week, randomized, placebo-controlled, double-blind study with 48 postmenopausal women with pre-hypertension or stage 1 hypertension investigated the effect of 22 grams of freeze-dried blueberry powder (1:1 highbush and rabbiteye), equivalent to a cup of fresh blueberries. After 8 weeks, both the mean systolic and diastolic blood pressures, as well as the brachial-ankle pulse wave velocity and nitric oxide blood levels, were significantly reduced compared to baseline values in the 25 patients of the blueberry group, but no significant changes occurred with the 23 control subjects.[54]

IN ANIMALS

Other evidence applicable to metabolic syndrome has been obtained from live animal studies, using combined blueberry species, lowbush blueberry, or uncharacterized blueberries. When freeze-dried blueberry powder (1:1 highbush and rabbiteye) was added as 4% weight to a high-fat diet in mice for 8 weeks, it attenuated or blocked a shift toward upregulation of inflammatory genes and a marker for oxidative stress and reduced glutathione peroxidase 3, compared to the high-fat diet alone. The blueberry diet also protected from high blood sugar and insulin resistance, along with reducing fat cell death.[55]

Freeze-dried skins of rabbiteye blueberries as 8% of the diet significantly reduced total cholesterol by 22% and VLDL-cholesterol by about 44% in hamsters fed a high-fat diet, while a comparable amount of the ethanol extract of these skins likewise reduced VLDL by 44% and total cholesterol by 29%, but additionally led to a significant 34% reduction in LDL-cholesterol. These blueberry diets increased excretion of lipids in the feces and upregulated liver CYP 7A1, indicative of increased bile acid synthesis, but fat cell inflammatory gene expression was not changed significantly.[56]

Freeze-dried lowbush blueberries fed as 1% of a diet to apolipo-protein E-deficient mice for 20 weeks significantly reduced the average atherosclerotic lesion area in the aortic sinus by 39% and descending aorta by 57% compared to controls. This occurred in spite of increases in total and LDL cholesterol in the mice fed blueberries, which also gained more weight due to their higher energy intake. The lipid peroxidation biomarker F_2-isoprostane was significantly lower in the liver of mice receiving blueberries, and the antioxidant enzymes superoxide dismutase and glutathione reductase were upregulated and showed significantly greater activity in the liver and/or serum of the blueberry-fed mice. Thus, oxidative stress reduction resulted in fewer lesions.[57]

Rats with normal blood pressure and spontaneously-hypertensive rats were compared with controls and each other when using diets of freeze-dried generic blueberries for 6 weeks (about 370 mg/day) or 12 weeks (about 400 mg/day, similar to 4.5 g daily of fresh berries). Those rats consuming the blueberries for 6 or 12 weeks had decreased blood pressure and renovascular resistance and improved kidney glomerular filtration rate. Kidney tissue showed lower oxidative stress indicators after long-term treatment and improved antioxidant status. This may possibly delay or modify hypertension-induced kidney damage.[58]

In a 10-week study with rats on regular or high fat and cholesterol diets known to induce endothelial dysfunction, groups on each diet were also supplemented with 2% freeze-dried highbush blueberry powder. Reductions in systolic blood pressure of 11% at 8 weeks and 14% at 10 weeks were observed with the regular diet plus blueberries, compared to controls without blueberries. On the high fat/cholesterol plus blueberry diet, systolic blood pressure was also reduced by 14% after 10 weeks, compared to high fat diet controls. Blueberry diets led to aortas harvested postmortem with reduced contractile responses to L-phenylephrine and greater relaxation from acetylcholine, compared to the controls on both diets.[59]

In studying weight gain in mice fed diets that were low-fat (10% of total calories from fat), high-fat (45% fat calories), or very high-fat (60% fat calories) diets, and comparing these control mice to low-fat and high-fat supplemented with 10% freeze-dried blueberries or very high-fat plus purified blueberry anthocyanin extract, blueberries did not alter glucose tolerance. In the high-fat diet with blueberries, weight gain and percent body fat increased significantly more than for high-fat controls after 8, 10, and 13 weeks. The very high-fat diet with anthocyanin extract had significantly lower weight gain and body fat than very high-fat controls after 7 weeks but not after 10 weeks.[60] However, studies in rodents bred to model human pathologies or fed artificial uniform diets not used by humans cannot be extrapolated with certainty to humans.

Preparations of wild lowbush blueberry were administered to diabetic mice by gavage to test for lowered blood sugar levels. Doses of 500 mg/kg body weight were given of either a concentrated phenol-rich methanolic extract providing 287 mg/g anthocyanins or an anthocyanin-enriched fraction delivering 595 mg/g of cyanidin 3-glucoside equivalents. Both were formulated with a self-microemulsifying drug delivery system called Labrasol, since no significant hypoglycemic effects were detected without Labrasol. With the Labrasol bio-enhancement, the anthocyanin fraction had greater hypoglycemic activity than the phenolic extract, indicating that anthocyanins are responsible for this effect. When 300 mg/kg doses of pure delphinidin-3-*O*-glucoside and malvidin-3-*O*-glucoside were compared, the malvidin anthocyanin was significantly hypoglycemic, but the delphinidin anthocyanin was not.[61]

IN VITRO

A freeze-dried ethanol extract of frozen lowbush blueberries was shown to significantly enhance proliferation of insulin-producing pancreatic beta-cells 2.8-fold and to reduce by 20-33% the apoptotic death of adrenal medullary PC12 cells exposed to elevated glucose for 96 hours.[62]

In testing for effects on the passage of oral hypoglycemic drugs through a dialysis tube, blueberry extract decreased permeation of metformin by only 20% but reduced that of glibenclamide by 45%, suggesting that the extract might modulate the absorption of these drugs somewhat *in vivo*.[63]

HEART AND VASCULAR EFFECTS

IN ANIMALS

Following a myocardial infarct (MI or heart attack), heart tissue damage is largely due to reactive oxygen species generated by lack of blood circulation to the cells. After feeding a diet with 20 g/kg freeze-dried blueberries or a control diet with 20 g/kg dried corn for 3 months to young rats and a coronary artery was tied off, the resulting MI was 22% less in those on the blueberry diet, and there were 40% less inflammatory cells (neutrophils and macrophages) in the area compared to controls. Ten weeks after the MI, the hearts of rats that continued on the blueberry diet recovered better than those taken off; even those switched to blueberry after the MI recovered better than controls.[64] The mortality over the next year was reduced 22% among the rats remaining on an isocaloric 2% blueberry extract diet. The heart ventricle maintained better integrity, and the MI expansion was arrested compared to controls.[65]

Compared to the control diet, rats fed a diet with 8% freeze-dried wild blueberries for 7 weeks showed a greater response to inhibition of nitric oxide synthase. In endothelium-dependent vasorelaxation induced by acetylcholine, involvement of nitric oxide pathways of the aorta was greater in mice fed blueberries. Vasoconstriction of the aortic rings by phenylephrine was reduced by the blueberry diet.[66]

POTENTIAL FOR REDUCING CANCER RISK

IN ANIMALS

Rats fed a control diet with or without 5% freeze-dried blueberries were injected with azoxymethane to induce aberrant crypt foci. Those receiving the blueberries had significantly fewer in the proximal colon compared to control diet only. The rats fed blueberries also had an average of 11 aberrant crypt foci in the entire colon, compared to an average of 172 in rats fed only the control diet (a 91% reduction), and significantly fewer total aberrant crypts (33) than rats who consumed 20% cranberry juice (165).[67] When rats were treated with the carcinogen N-nitrosomethylbenzylamine (NMBA) for 5 weeks and then placed on a diet with 5% freeze-dried blueberries, the berry diet significantly reduced tumorigenesis in the rat esophagus, both in incidence (33% less) and multiplicity. In addition, serum interleukin (IL)-5, cytokines, and other oxidation markers were reduced, while serum antioxidant capacity increased.[68]

In a study of female rats given a 17β-estradiol implant to induce tumors of the mammary glands, the animals were given a control diet with or without 5% freeze-dried organic blueberries. Tumor appearance occurred in controls at 84 days, but this was significantly delayed by 24 days with the blueberry diet. The blueberry diet also reduced mammary tissue proliferation and tumor burden. Blueberries significantly reduced cytochrome P-450 (CYP) 1A1 expression involved with estradiol conversion.[69] CYP expression and phase II metabolic enzymes bear important roles in estrogen's carcinogenic effects.

In a prior study of the rats given the estrogen implant, a control diet or diets with 1% or 2.5% blueberry were given 2 weeks before the estrogen and 6, 18, or 24 weeks afterward. After 6 weeks, the implanted controls had a 48-fold increase in CYP1A1 that was significantly attenuated to 21-fold by the 2.5% blueberry diet, and this diet also significantly reduced CYP1B1 expression by 6-fold. The 5-fold induction of 17β-hydroxysteroid dehydrogenase was significantly reduced to about 2-fold by the 2.5% supplemented berry diet after 6 weeks. After 18 weeks, the blueberry diet reduced the estrogen induction of CYP1A1, in this case from 15-fold down to 7-fold and reversed the 2-fold induction of catechol-O-methyl transferase expression. At 24 weeks, the CYP1A1 induction was not reduced by the blueberry diet. The 1% and 2.5% blueberry diets reduced mammary tumor incidence 0% and 31%, tumor multiplicity 2.6% and 38%, and tumor volume 41% and 59%, respectively, probably by suppressing estrogen-metabolizing enzymes early in estrogen-induced carcinogenesis.[70]

In female nude mice, triple negative (no expression of ER, PR, or HER2 protein) breast tumor volume was reduced 75% by a 5% freeze-dried blueberry diet compared to controls. Tumor cell proliferation was also significantly reduced, and expression of genes important for inflammation, cancer, and metastasis were also significantly altered, e.g., IL-13, IFNγ, and Wnt signaling. The 5% diet also significantly reduced liver metastasis by 70% and lymph node metastasis by 25% compared to controls.[71]

Giving a freeze-dried hydroethanolic blueberry extract orally to mice with hemangioendothelioma significantly reduced tumor size at 10-20 mg/kg body weight and significantly increased survival time at 20 mg/kg. Studies on the endothelial precursor cells *in vitro* showed that the extract is both antiangiogenic and inhibits both c-Jun N-terminal kinase (JNK) and nuclear factor-kappa B (NFκB) signalling pathways associated with tumor formation. This could potentially be applicable to children with endothelial cell neoplasms, the most common soft-tissue tumors in infants.[72]

Pterostilbene, a phenolic compound found in blueberries, when given for 8 weeks at 40 parts per million in the diet of rats exposed twice to azoxymethane, significantly reduced by 57% the aberrant crypt foci induced in the colon by azoxymethane. Multiple clusters of aberrant crypts were likewise significantly reduced 29% by pterostilbene. The suppression azoxymethane-induced colonic cell proliferation may be of use in helping to prevent colon cancer.[73]

A diet with 2% blueberries given to rats for 8 weeks prior to exposure to 1.5 or 2.0 Gy accelerated iron particles produced significantly better performance on behavioral tasks compared to control rats. It also reduced the tumorigenesis induced by the heavy particles 1 year after exposure, compared to controls.[74]

In Vitro

A methanolic extract of blueberries was tested in several human tumor cell lines for antiproliferative activity in comparison with 5 other berries (cranberry, strawberry, and 3 *Rubus* spp.). The extract was moderately effective against oral and breast cancer cell cultures, but was especially active against colon (surpassed by blackberry and black raspberry) and prostate cancer cells (at IC_{50} of 36.5 mcg/ml surpassing all other berries).[75]

When rabbiteye cultivar extracts and fractions were tested in 2 colon cancer cell lines, the anthocyanin fraction was most active with >50% inhibition at 15-50 mg/ml, close to the concentration range of anthocyanins found in rat plasma, followed by IC_{50} of the tannin fraction of 50-100 mcg/ml and of the flavonol fraction of 70-100 mcg/ml. The anthocyanin fraction also increased cancer cell DNA framentation 2-7 times, indicative of induced apoptosis.[76]

The phenolic acid fraction of rabbiteye blueberries reduced liver cancer HepG2 cell line 50% at 1-2 mg/ml, while the anthocyanin fraction produced the same effect at the lower 70-150 mcg/ml concentration, and flavonol and tannin fractions were intermediate. The anthocyanin fraction also resulted in a 2- to 4-fold increase in DNA fragmentation, showing its induction of cancer cell apoptosis, and indication that blueberries may help reduce liver cancer risk.[77]

In comparing fractions of hydroacetonic extracts from quick-frozen wild blueberries and cultivated blueberries for inhibitory effects on androgen-sensitive human prostate cancer cell line LNCaP, the proanthocyanidin fraction 5 of the wild blueberries was the most potent at 20 mcg/ml, reducing growth to 11% of controls, while at this concentration both proanthocyanidin fractions 4 and 5 of cultivated blueberries were significantly more effective at reducing growth than controls (57% and 26%, respectively). Only fraction 5 of cultivated blueberries significantly inhibited the androgen-insensitive cell line DU145.[78]

On the other hand, lowbush blueberry crude methanolic extract, hydromethanolic fraction, and hydroacetonic fraction were all effective in down-regulating matrix metalloproteinases (MMPs) in DU145 human prostate cancer cells by multiple mechanisms. MMPs are crucial in regulating metastasis.[79] Extracts of lowbush blueberry fruit showed that oligomeric proanthocyanidin-rich fractions were both anti-proliferative for human prostate cancer and mouse liver cancer cell lines.[80]

A depectinized, flavonoid-rich acetone extract of juice from lowbush blueberries was shown to induce the phase II enzyme quinone reductase without having cytotoxicity, indicating its potential for inhibiting the initial stage of carcinogenesis.[18] Besides doubling quinone reductase activity by lowbush blueberry ethyl acetate fraction at 4.2 mcg tannic acid equivalents (TAE), the crude methanolic extract at 8.0 mcg TAE and the polymeric proanthocyanidin fraction at 3.0 mcg TAE inhibited by 50% the ornithine decarboxylase activity induced by the tumor promoter phorbol 12-myristate 13-acetate (TPA).[81]

IMPROVING MUSCLE RECOVERY, REDUCING PAIN AND PREVENTING RADIATION DAMAGE

IN HUMANS

To test whether blueberries given before and after intensive exercise would reduce the recovery time and oxidative stress response resulting from the muscle damage, 10 women were studied in a randomized, placebo-controlled, cross-over design. A serving of 200 grams of blueberries in a smoothy, or a placebo isocaloric- and antioxidant-equivalent smoothy without the blueberries, was given 5 and 10 hours before strenuous eccentric contractions of the quadriceps, then immediately after, and 12 and 36 hours after the exercise. The biggest difference in the two drinks was a much higher phenolic content (168 mg vs. 29 mg), especially anthocyanins (97 mg vs. 0), in the blueberry smoothie. Performance measurements were taken at 12, 36, and 60 hours after the exercise.[82]

A significant interaction with blueberry and faster rate of recovery for peak isometric tension in the first 36-hour recovery period was measured. Other trends of better muscle strength recovery for concentric and eccentric torque were also seen. A significant decrease in oxidative stress in the blueberry group until 36 hours post-exercise coincided with increased plasma antioxidant capacity. Thus, the blueberry beverage appeared to up-regulate the adaptive processes following muscle damage from exercise.[82]

IN ANIMALS

An anthocyanin extract of freeze-dried rabbiteye blueberries was given orally to mice at 3.2 mg/kg or 6.4 mg/kg daily for 21 days or as a single treatment and was compared to water controls, morphine, and the NSAID diclofenac to assess its pain-reducing activity. Pain induced by acetic acid was significantly reduced with long-term and single use at both doses, compared to controls, but was less effective than morphine after one use. Formalin pain inhibition was graded, being as effective as diclofenac with long- and short-term use, but less effective than morphine after one treatment. Hot-plate and tail-flick tests showed that prolonged rabbiteye blueberry extract treatment significantly increased the pain threshold of mice compared to water, while a single higher dose extract treatment was slower but as effective as 10 mg morphine.[83]

When a blueberry extract was given as 2% of the diet for 2 months to rats that were then exposed to high doses of radiation, the extract prevented deterioration in performance of cognitive, spatial learning and memory tasks compared to rats on a control diet. The damage from radiation is similar to the effects of aging, based on free radical generation and antioxidant stress. A year after the radiation, the rats on the extract diet had significantly fewer tumors induced by the radiation than those on the control diet.[84]

When a blueberry extract was given as 2% of the diet for 2 months to rats that were then exposed to high doses of radiation, the extract prevented deterioration in performance of cognitive, spatial learning and memory tasks compared to rats on a control diet.[84]

BLADDER PROTECTION

IN VITRO

It is well-known and demonstrated that cranberry juice prevents attachment of uropathic *E. coli* to mucosal cells by inhibiting the bacterial adhesin MR. Of 6 other juices tested (cranberry, plus blueberry, grapefruit, guava, mango, orange, and pineapple), only blueberry juice also produced this inhibitory effect.[80] Tests on lowbush blueberry extracts showed that oligomeric proanthocyanidin-rich fractions were anti-adhesive for *E. coli*.[85]

PROCESSING AND STORAGE EFFECTS ON PHYTOCHEMICALS AND ANTIOXIDANT ACTIVITY

FRESH

Fresh blueberries should be picked when fully blue and firm, and several picking are necessary as the berries ripen at different rates. After poor quality berries are culled, the berries should be forced-air cooled within an hour after picking to as near freezing (0 °C; 32 °F) as possible, as well as while stored and displayed. In addition, 10%-15% CO_2, 1%-10% O_2, and relative humidity above 90% during the first several weeks while kept at or below 5 °C (41 °F) are optimal for extending storage up to 6 weeks, as controlling atmospheric conditions is very important. Bruising reduces shelf-life of fresh berries, so compared to hand harvesting, mechanical harvesting can reduce storage life by about half. Postharvest berries may be subject to ripe rot (*Colletotrichum gloesosporiodes*), while damaged berries are quite susceptible to gray mold (*Botyris cinerea*) growth that is stimulated in the presence of ethylene. Methyl bromide fumigation is used to control blueberry maggot (*Rhagoletis mendax*) postharvest infestation during long-distance transport.[86] Sulfur dioxide fumigation is also used to decrease decay and extend market life.

When fresh highbush blueberries were dipped for 15-30 seconds in water at 22 °C (room temperature) or 45, 50, or 60 °C (hot), dried and then stored for 4 weeks at 0 °C, the hotter the water treatment, the greater percentage of marketable berries (90%-83%), compared to controls (76%). Likewise, after 2 additional days of storage at 20 °C, decay incidence was reduced (0.6%-2.8%) by hot water from control levels (5.1%), while after 7 more days decay with 60 °C water exposure for 15 seconds was 1.8% compared to controls at 37.4%. Weight loss, shriveled and split berries were significantly reduced by hot water treatment, and yeast and mold counts were reduced by 30 second treatment. There was no effect on firmness, pH, or most flavor volatiles.[87]

The antioxidant capacity of fresh highbush and lowbush blueberries strongly correlated with total phenolics and anthocyanin contents which were higher in lowbush berries, but ascorbate was higher in highbush berries. After 8 days of fresh storage at 0, 10, 20, or 30 °C, the only significant changes in these parameters were anthocyanin content of highbush berries that was higher at 20 °C, while the ascorbate content of lowbush berries was lower at 20 and 30 °C.[88] At 5 °C various cultivars of fresh blueberry were successfully stored at marketable quality for <3 weeks up to 7 weeks, depending on the cultivar. None showed a significant decrease from the antioxidant activity at harvest. Fruit maturity correlated significantly with antioxidant activity and total phenolic and anthocyanin contents, and some cultivars had increases in one or more of these during cold storage.[89]

FROZEN

Highbush blueberries were frozen for 1 month or 3 months at -20 °C and then compared with the same blueberries either fresh or fresh but stored for 2 weeks at 5 °C, in regards to the total anthocyanin content and antioxidant effect. While the anthocyanin contents of 2-week stored fresh berries were lower (5.7 mg/g dried) than the levels of fresh blueberries (7.2 mg/g), the frozen samples had higher anthocyanin contents after 1 month (8.1 mg/g) and 3 months (7.9 mg/g), though none of these differences were significant. Likewise, the antioxidant activities in reducing the 2, 2-diphenyl-1-picrylhydrazyl (DPPH) radical between the 2 fresh and 2 frozen berry samples did not differ significantly.[90]

> While the anthocyanin contents of 2-week stored fresh berries were lower (5.7 mg/g dried) than the levels of fresh blueberries (7.2 mg/g), the frozen samples had higher anthocyanin contents after 1 month (8.1 mg/g). [90]

FREEZE-DRIED

In comparing freeze-dried blueberries with fresh fruit, ascorbic acid (vitamin C) was significantly decreased in the freeze-dried berries. However, in vacuum freeze-dried blueberries the total polyphenols were increased significantly when treated with infrared light, so that there was no significant difference in the antioxidant efficiency with the fresh berries.[91] When freeze-dried blueberries were compared to the frozen berries, there was a small reduction in anthocyanin content of 3.9%, but a large 1.9-fold increase on average in phenolic acids.[15]

> When freeze-dried blueberries were compared to the frozen berries, there was a small reduction in anthocyanin content of 3.9%, but a large 1.9-fold increase on average in phenolic acids.[15]

When storing freeze-dried wild lowbush blueberry powder for 7 weeks at 25, 42, 60, and 80 °C, the total and single anthocyanin content and total antioxidant activities were compared. Storage reduced all anthocyanin levels, the slowest reduction of -3% occurring at 25 °C after 2 weeks, whereas at 80 °C after 3 days there was rapid reductions of -80%. Half-life estimates for anthocyanins were 139 days at 25 °C, 39 days at 42 °C, and 12 days at 60 °C. However, the total antioxidant activity was not affected significantly by increased temperature.[92] Nonetheless, it appears evident that storing freeze-dried blueberries at lower temperatures helps preserve the phytochemical integrity and associated broad bioactivity.

DRIED

When compared with highbush blueberries frozen for 1 month or 3 months at -20 °C and with fresh blueberries, berries that were cabinet-dried had a significant reduction of 41% in total anthocyanins. In comparison with the anthocyanin content of fresh berries of 7.2 mg/g, the dried blueberry anthocyanins amounted to only 4.3 mg/g. However, the antioxidant activity of anthocyanin extracts of the fresh, frozen, and dried blueberries were not significantly different, when measured by reducing DPPH radical concentration.[90]

When compared with highbush blueberries frozen for 1 month or 3 months at -20 °C and with fresh blueberries, berries that were cabinet-dried had a significant reduction of 41% in total anthocyanins.[90]

CANNED

The effects of processing after the first day and after storage for 1, 3, and 6 months on anthocyanin content and oxygen radical absorbance capacity (ORAC) was compared between 1-month frozen highbush blueberries and the same batch of frozen berries after canning. Fully ripe frozen berries in cans were covered in either boiling water or a water/corn syrup mixture, placed in a steam box for 4 minutes before sealing, then immersed in boiling water for 15 minutes, and stored at 25 °C.[93] After 1 day, the total monomeric anthocyanin losses in the berries in syrup was less than in water, -28% vs. -34%,[93] but procyanidin reductions were -35% in the syrup berries and only -22% in the water berries.[94]

Over the 6 month span, a similar percentage of total anthocyanin monomers was found in the fluid syrup medium (14% to 23%) as for the water medium (17% to 23%). With steady declines in each type over time, in canned blueberries after 6 months of storage the change in monomeric anthocyanins for berries in syrup was -71% compared to -62% for berries in water.[93] The decline in procyanidins was -78% for berries in syrup versus -68% for those in water.[94] While the ORAC in the syrup- and water-canned berries were initially reduced by -46% and -42%, respectively, the levels during storage were fairly stable, though from 1 to 6 months an additional -12% loss was found in the syrup berries. The anthocyanin polymers formed during storage apparently retained much of the antioxidant activity found originally in the monomers. Overall, the blueberries canned in water had superior monomeric anthocyanin retention and antioxidant capacity than those in syrup,[93] as well as better procyanidin retention.[94]

In canned blueberries after 6 months of storage the change in monomeric anthocyanins for berries in syrup was -71% compared to -62% for berries in water.[93]

Canned highbush blueberries were prepared similarly with a syrup medium using organically and conventionally grown berries from 2 different types of cultivars, and then stored at room temperature (23 °C) for up to 13 months. After this time, the total anthocyanins, total phenolics, and total antioxidant activity in the unblanched canned berries changed by -86%, -69%, and -52%, respectively, whereas the total antioxidant activity loss was only -7% in blanched berries. Blanching blueberries before they are thermally processed also was shown to preserve the anthocyanins during storage (65% retention after 13 months, compared to only 33% retained without blanching). The losses of anthocyanins and antioxidant activity in the syrup were -68% and -15%, respectively. These results for both cultivars did not depend on whether the blueberries were organically or conventionally grown.[95]

PUREES AND BAKING

The effects of storage on day 1 and after 1, 3, and 6 months was compared for anthocyanins and ORAC between highbush blueberries frozen 1-month and the same batch of frozen berries that were pureed. Thawed blueberries were homogenized and heated to 95 °C, and corn syrup was added. The mixture was added to jars, sealed, and boiled for 15 minutes, then cooled and stored in the dark at 25 °C.[93]

The pureed berries had an initial -43% change in total anthocyanin monomers compared to original levels in the frozen berries and continued to diminish to -48% after 1 month, -67% after 3 months, and -80% after 6 months. This, in conjunction with increased polymeric color values, indicates extensive polymerization during storage. Pureeing led to a loss of -47% in antioxidant capacity, but this remained fairly stable during storage though a further -9% change occurred between 1 and 6 months.[93] For procyanidin components, 41% were retained after initial processing. Following 6 months of storage, all that remained was 7%.[94] On the other hand, it was found that blanching highbush blueberries before making a puree led to significantly higher maximum anthocyanin absorption and a higher phenolic content of the plasma after consumption by healthy human subjects.[96]

The pureed berries had an initial -43% change in total anthocyanin monomers compared to original levels in the frozen berries and continued to diminish to -48% after 1 month, -67% after 3 months, and -80% after 6 months.[93]

Tests were performed on freeze-dried lowbush blueberry powder, mixing the powder in 40 grams of bun dough and proving at 30 °C, cooking the berry powder in 20 grams of filling at 90 °C, and baking them together at 180 °C for 12 minutes. These processes reduced anthocyanin levels and increased chlorogenic acid, while quercetin and caffeic and ferulic acid levels were constant. Total procyanidins did not change with these processes, but high molecular weight oligomers decreased and lower molecular weight procyanidins increased.[97] In regard to resveratrol loss, highbush blueberries from Michigan, rabbiteye blueberries from Mississippi, and lowbush blueberries from Nova Scotia were obtained raw. The highbush and lowbush berries showed reductions of 46% and 26%, respectively, when baked at 190 °C for 18 minutes as they would be in muffins. Resveratrol could not be detected in the rabbiteye blueberries.[5]

JUICE

In production of blueberry juice the yield was 83% by weight, but only 32% of the anthocyanins were retained. The amount of anthocyanins remaining in the berry press-cake residue was 18%. Other berry content recovered in the juice includes 35% of flavonols, 43% of procyanidins, and 53% of chlorogenic acid. The large loss of anthocyanins and other polyphenolics during processing was believed to be due to polyphenol oxidase in the berries. Further losses during concentration of the juice included 20% of procyanidins. The profile of anthocyanins was greatly altered, with delphinidin glycosides being the least stable and malvidin glycosides the most stable.[98]

In production of blueberry juice the yield was 83% by weight, but only 32% of the anthocyanins were retained.[98]

The effects of storage on anthocyanin and ORAC after 1 day and 1, 3, and 6 months was compared between highbush blueberries frozen 1-month versus clarified and nonclarified juice from the same batch of frozen berries. After blanching for 3 minutes at 95 °C, the enzymatically depectinized berries were pressed and half of the juice was clarified by centrifugation. Both juices were bottled in glass and some of each was heated to 90 °C for pasteurization. All were capped and stored at 25 °C in the dark. Compared to the frozen berries after 1 day, the non-clarified non-pasteurized juice and non-clarified pasteurized juice had significantly less monomeric anthocyanins and lower ORAC, but significantly more anthocyanins and higher ORAC when compared to clarified, non-pasturized juice and clarified, pasteurized juice.[93]

This demonstrates that clarifying the juice initially produced a greater diminishment in anthocyanin and antioxidant capacity than pasteurization. Pasteuriation caused only minor alterations of these parameters, though all forms of juice were significantly diminished compared to frozen berries. In addition, pasteurized juice retained anthocyanins following 1, 3, and 6 months of storaged better than non-pasteurized juice. After 6 months of storage, clarified and non-clarified unpasteurized juices retained only 15% and 23%, respectively, of the original anthocyanins.[93] A similar but greater degradation was shown with procyanidins, with only 19% and 23% initially retained in clarified and non-clarified juices, respectively, and these were reduced after 6 months of storage to 8% for clarified and 11% for non-clarified juice compared to procyanidins found in the frozen blueberries.

However, for procyanidins the losses from pasteurization were greater than from clarification.[96]

Clarifying the juice initially produced a
greater diminishment in anthocyanin and
antioxidant capacity than pasteurization.[93]

Another study using 2 cultivars of rabbiteye blueberries prepared an extract from frozen berries by thawing, blanching, milling, treating with pectinase, centrifuging, collecting the supernatant, heating to 85 °C, then cooling to 30 °C and storing in glass bottles. This is equivalent to a clarified and pasteurized juice. After pressing and heating the extract, the total polyphenols, total anthocyanins, and Trolox equivalent antioxidant capacity (TEAC) recovered were about 25%, 29%, and 65%, respectively. For individual anthocyanidin of both cultivars, malvidin and cyanidin glucosides recovered were about 22%, whereas for peonidin glucoside and arabinoside it was about 55%. After storing the extracted juice at -20, 6, 23, and 35 °C for up to 60 days, the further phytochemical losses were progressive but less than the initial losses from processing. Freezing and storage at low temperatures are best for preserving bioactive components.[99]

In still another study non-clarified pasteurized juice from blanched and non-blanched highbush blueberries was stored for 4 months at 23 °C. After storage, total anthocyanins changed by -64% to -82% with blanching and -74% to -79% without blanching, while total phenols increased 28% to 30% without blanching and 15% to 25% with blanching. Blanching reduced the losses in total juice antioxidant activity during storage of -26% to -30% and brought them down to -21% to -22%. Blanching acts by reducing enzymatic degradation and/or improving extraction on phenolics. So, decreases in anthocyanins and antioxidant activity after juice storage were smaller when the berries were blanched beforehand.[95]

DRIED EXTRACTS

Five dehydrated extract products of blueberry (and 11 such extracts of bilberry) sold as commercial dietary supplements in the forms of tablets (2 products), soft capsules (2 products), and granules (1 product) were obtained and tested for anthocyanin deterioration using ultra-high performance liquid chromatography, along with assessing the thermal stability. After exposure to 70 °C for 5 days, the increases in anthocyanidins was mirrored by a decrease in anthocyanins. The increase in the degradation index due to thermal breakdown was greater for blueberry granules than for bilberry soft capsules that was likewise greater than for bilberry tablets. The degradation index for anthocyanins in different blueberry extracts showed that the breakdowns during storage in granules were also higher than for tablets and soft capsules. This study illustrates that anthocyanin degradation occurs in dried blueberry extracts, as it does in blueberry juice.[100]

Anthocyanin degradation occurs in dried blueberry extracts, as it does in blueberry juice.[100]

JAMS

Fresh blueberries made into jams were tested for polyphenolic content and antioxidant activity immediately after processing and during storage for 6 months at 4 °C and 25 °C. Jam processing and storage resulted in large losses of anthocyanins and procyanidins and decreases of chlorogenic acid, while ORAC was lowered during processing, but flavonols were retained well during both. Storage at 4°C led to fewer losses than at room temperature, indicative of the benefits of refrigerating jams to maintain polyphenolic content and antioxidant capacity.[101]

Jam processing and storage resulted in large losses of anthocyanins and procyanidins.[101]

EFFECTS OF PROCESSING

Fresh blueberries have a shelf life of only several weeks when refrigerated, whereas frozen berries maintain their value for months. Freeze-dried blueberries kept at low temperature offer the best prospect for long-term storage. Processing of fresh and frozen blueberries results in significant reductions in monomeric anthocyanins and antioxidant capacity. Further degradations occur during storage in all heat-processed products, including canned blueberries, purees, and juices, resulting after 6 months in less than 40% of the total anthocyanins initially in the processed products. Since polymerization of the monomeric anthocyanins occurs during storage, smaller losses in antioxidant capacity occur. For canned berries 14% to 25% of anthocyanins are leached into the water or syrup.[93] Procyanidin losses were generally even greater, both after initial processing and after 6 months.[94] Blanching the blueberries helps preserve the phytochemicals and antioxidant activity in whole canned berries more than for the juice.[95] Dried blueberry extracts taken as dietary supplements are subject to undergoing greater degradation at higher temperatures,[100] much like the blueberry jam.[101]

SUMMARY

Though blueberry species and cultivars vary in amounts of anthocyanins, proanthocyanidins, and stilbenes, they all contain these potent free radical scavengers that provide protection from oxidative stress. Processing or storage that involves exposure to heat diminishes phenolic content. Importantly, the anthocyanin antioxidants penetrate the blood-brain barrier and help preserve nerve integrity, especially as it applies to aging and memory. In the cardiovascular system and beyond, blueberry polyphenolics can help reduce the trend toward atherosclerosis, high blood pressure, and type 2 diabetes that are associated with the growing scourge of metabolic syndrome. Likewise, to help reduce the tendency toward cancer initiation, the inclusion of blueberries in the diet adds important components that may help protect against damage from radiation and carcinogens. Since heating leads to a breakdown of bioactive blueberry components, research findings support the preferred consumption of fresh, frozen, and/or freeze-dried blueberries.

Cranberry

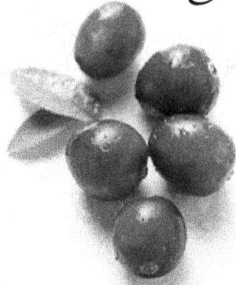

WHILE CRANBERRY HAS LONG BEEN CONSUMED AS PART OF THE AMERICAN THANKSGIVING CELEBRATION IN NOVEMBER, OVER THE LAST 50 YEARS ITS JUICE HAS ALSO BEEN POPULAR FOR HELPING PREVENT URINARY TRACT INFECTIONS (UTIs). MORE RECENT RESEARCH DEMONSTRATES THAT ITS USEFULNESS EXTENDS BEYOND BEING A TANGY SEASONAL TREAT OR A LOCALLY BENEFICIAL BEVERAGE. THE ANTI-ADHESION EFFECTS OF THIS BERRY ON PATHOGENIC BACTERIA AFFECTING MUCOSA CAN ALSO IMPACT THE GASTROINTESTINAL TRACT. IN ADDITION, THE ANTIOXIDANT ACTIVITY YIELDS SYSTEMIC ADVANTAGES FOR THE CARDIOVASCULAR SYSTEM, ESPECIALLY FOR THOSE WITH PROBLEMS ASSOCIATED WITH METABOLIC SYNDROME, AS WELL AS PROVIDING CHEMOPREVENTIVE POTENTIAL. THIS RED COUSIN OF THE BLUEBERRIES YIELDS SIMILAR COMPONENTS AND FAMILIAR TRAITS.

ANTIOXIDANT CONTENT AND BIOAVAILABILITY

The potent antioxidant activity of cranberry (*Vaccinium macrocarpon*) anthocyanins (peonidin- and cyanidin-3-galactoside, -arabinoside, and -glucoside) along with its flavonols (quercetin, myricetin), flavan-3-ols (proanthocyanidins, epicatechin), phenolic acids (benzoic, coumaric, sinapic, caffeic, and ellagic acids) and stilbene (resveratrol) holds promise for helping lower the risk of chronic disease.[1,2] Based on fresh weight, the free and total phenols in mg/g cranberries decrease in concentration in commercial products going from powdered to dried to frozen to whole berry sauce to jellied sauce, and in mg/ml in beverages from juice to juice mixtures to juice cocktail to white juice.[3] Cranberries are also high in antioxidant carotenes especially when fresh, as compared by weight to the dried sweetened berries or the juice or juice cocktail.[2] Heat and oxygen, along with light and alkalinity, destabilize anthocyanin content of cranberry juice.[4]

The content of proanthocyanidins (PACs), also called condensed tannins, in raw berries is much greater than in the juice or juice cocktail. Procyanidins, a subclass of PACs, are a mixture of linked catechin and epicatechin units which in cranberry consist largely of epicatechin. Unlike most other foods, the procyanidins in cranberry are linked via A-type bonds that are responsible for the unique anti-adhesion action.[2] It is these PACs in cranberry that are primarily credited with its helping prevent UTIs, since the juice and its organic acids fail to adequately lower urine pH as once was believed.[1,5]

> Unlike most other foods, the procyanidins in cranberry are linked via A-type bonds that are responsible for the unique anti-adhesion action.[2]

The greatest phytochemical difference between cranberry juice, cranberry water extracts, and the whole cranberry is the vastly higher content of the triterpenoids ursolic acid and its ester found in the whole berry. Fresh *V. macrocarpon* cultivars contain from 0.05% to 0.1% ursolic acid, while *V. oxycoccus* has only 1/4 to 1/8 this amount. Whole dried cranberry powder has from 0.85% to 1.37% ursolic acid.[6] When the phytochemical content and radical scavenging activity of ethanolic extracts of 4 cranberry cultivar presscakes (berry material left after juice is expressed) and of the whole berries were compared, presscake extracts radical scavenging activity were only slightly less than for whole berry extracts, while phenolic and anthocyanin content of presscake extracts were greater, likely due to greater presscake content of berry skins.[7] The lack of ursolic acid in cranberry juice and high phenolic content of the berry presscakes illustrates the phytochemical advantage of consuming whole cranberries over juice.

IN HUMANS

The main phenolic metabolites are cyanidin- and peonidin-3-glycosides,[4,7] hippuric acid, salicyluric and dihydroxybenzoic acids, and quercetin glucuronide.[5] Most cranberry phenolic compounds and/or their metabolites have been found to be bioavailable in the plasma or excreted in the urine.[4] A single dose given to 10 healthy adults over the age of 50 years, using a low-calorie cocktail with 54% cranberry juice, showed individual variability with different compounds. The total antioxidant capacity of the plasma correlated with the peaks of certain phenolic metabolites after 30 minutes and again after 6-8 hours. The first plasma peaks for most phenolic acids, flavanols, and flavonols appeared in 0.5-2.6 hours, in concentrations substantially higher than similar timed peaks for anthocyanins. Total phenolic bioavailability in the plasma followed a bimodal pattern, reaching a second peak level of 34.2 mcg/ml between 8-10 hours, but the anthocyanins were absent at this time. Urinary peaks for total phenolics occurred 2-4 hours earlier than for plasma. PAC-A2 dimers in the urine rose to a maximum of 24.4 ng at 11 hours and diminished gradually over the next 14 hours.[8]

USE FOR URINARY TRACT CONDITIONS

Cranberry products have been effective for preventing UTIs range in forms from the liquid cranberry juice to the juice cocktail and from solid spray-dried juice to cranberry tablets or encapsulated fruit powder.[1] An advantage of cranberry powder in capsules or tablets is avoidance of the intake of necessary sweeteners added to the juice cocktail.[2]

An advantage of cranberry powder in capsules or tablets is avoidance of the intake of necessary sweeteners added to the juice cocktail.[2]

IN HUMANS

Consumption of cranberry for health has been mostly associated with using its juice to lower the risk of urinary tract infections (UTIs). UTIs are 50 times more common in women than men, so that about

50% of women will have one or more UTI in their lifetime, accounting for over 7 million physician office visits for this condition each year.[1] Daily consumption of 300 ml of the juice high in organic acids such as quinic, malic and citric acids reduces the amount of bacteria and white blood cells in the urine significantly after 2 months. However, besides added sweetener, cranberry juice has lost much of the nutritional content in the berries,[9] as shown in the high phenolic content of presscakes after juice extraction.[7]

A study on asymptomatic bacteriuria in 188 pregnant women randomized them to 240 ml low-calorie (sucralose-sweetened) cranberry juice cocktail (27% cranberry juice with 106 mg PACs) 2-3 times daily (n=58), placebo 2-3 times daily (n=63), or cranberry once and then placebo twice daily (n=67) with meals. Among those who completed the study compliance was poor and use lasted about 6 months, while about 39% (n=73) dropped out after about 2 months due in part to nausea, vomiting, diarrhea, or dislike of taste (n=44). There was a trend for fewer asymptomatic and symptomatic UTIs among those who used multiple cranberry doses, but less so for the single cranberry dose group, than for those taking only placebo, but the differences were not significant. There were no differences in obstetrical or neonatal outcomes between groups.[10]

In a 2008 Cochrane Review of ten studies of good methodology using cranberry products to prevent UTIs with 1049 total subjects, 5 were crossover studies and 5 were parallel-group studies. Seven compared cranberry juice with water, juice or placebo, while 3 used cranberry tablets compared to placebo. The durations ranged from 1 to 12 months, while 5 studies lasted 6 months. Half of the studies showed a decreased incidence of UTIs with cranberry use, with results more effective for women than in the elderly. However, due to the different products, doses, and durations reviewed, no absolute judgement can be rendered on the basis of this review.[11] The results appear to be different when used during a UTI rather than for prevention. A 2011 placebo-controlled, double-blind study of 319 college women treated for acute UTI found no difference in the recurrence rate over 6 months of those taking 8 oz twice daily of a 27% cranberry juice than those using placebo.[12]

When 12 women who had 6 UTIs in the previous year were given cranberry extract capsules twice daily for 12 weeks to provide about 100 mg per day of total PACs, none developed a UTI during that time (when a total of 24 UTIs would have been expected). Eight continued with various cranberry products for 2 years with no recurrences of UTIs, while four stopped taking cranberry supplements. Of those who stopped, two developed symptoms that resolved with resumption of cranberry products, and one had a UTI treated with antibiotics but resumed cranberry use and had no further symptoms.[13] When 8 oz (240 ml) of cranberry juice cocktail was given with the oral beta-lactam antibiotics amoxicillin and cefaclor, used to treat resistant organisms in recurrent UTIs, there was no significant effect on the oral absorption or renal clearance of the antibiotics.[14]

Effects can vary when using different forms. Women with at least 3 UTIs in the prior 6 months were randomized in groups of 37 and given in a double-blind fashion within 6 hours of sexual intercourse (at least once every 2 weeks) either whole cranberry powder, cranberry extract with 36 mg PAC-A, or placebo. Those receiving whole cranberry powder had the lowest recurrent cystitis episode rate after 45 days: 10.8% for the powder, compared to 18.9% for the extract and 43.2% for placebo. The average number of days prior to the first infection was also less for the powder (22 days), compared to the extract (8 days) and placebo (4 days), independent of the first incidence of intercourse (2 days on average for each group) or average number of sexual relations prior to symptoms (12.3, 8.4 and 11.5, respectively).[15]

Those receiving whole cranberry powder had the lowest recurrent cystitis episode rate after 45 days: 10.8% for the powder, compared to 18.9% for the extract and 43.2% for placebo.[15]

In 20 women with recurrent UTIs (2 within the past 6 months and/or at least 3 within the last year), a 42 gram serving of sweetened dried cranberries was consumed once daily for 2 weeks. In comparison with the number of UTIs in the prior 6 months, there was a significant reduction in the UTI rate in the 6 months after consuming the dried cranberries. Also, the time until the first UTI after beginning consumption was significantly greater, compared to a previous group of control patients.[16]

In another study of UTI recurrence, 213 women of ages 20-79 years participated; 188 had multiple recurrences within the prior year. Of these subjects, 107 consumed a 125 ml bottle of cranberry juice once daily at bedtime for 24 weeks, while the others drank a placebo beverage. Of the 118 over the age of 50 years with acute uncomplicated cystitis, significantly fewer (29.1%) who used cranberry juice had a relapse, compared to the 49.2% who relapsed taking placebo.[17]

In 20 women of average age of 35.2 years with recurrent postcoital urinary tract infections, a sachet of cranberry extract yielding 118 mg of PACs was given once daily for 3 days after their first sexual intercourse in a week, then they received one sachet only on the day after the second and subsequent sexual encounters. If symptoms occurred during the first 2 days after intercourse, they received antibiotic treatment. The number of infections in the 3 months prior to taking the extract averaged 2.8, but with cranberry extract this was significantly reduced to 0.7 after 3 months and 0.2 after 6 months, an improvement of 93%. At baseline, all 20 had infections with positive urine cultures for *Escherichia coli*, but after 6 months only 3 had symptomatic infections, 2 of which were *E. coli*. Quality of life rating assessments significantly improved from 62.4 at baseline to 78.2 after 6 months, a 20% improvement.[18]

In a randomized, controlled, double-blind study with 137 women over 45 years of age who had 2 or more urinary tract infections treated with antibiotics in the previous 12 months, 69 used 500 mg of cranberry extract while 68 took 100 mg of the antibiotic trimethoprim at bedtime for 6 months. During this period after 17 withdrawals due to adverse effects (6 from cranberry and 11 from trimethoprim), 25 in the cranberry group and 14 in the antibiotic group had another antibiotic-treated urinary tract infection. Though trimethoprim was more effective, the difference in relative risk was not significant, and cranberry had fewer adverse effects. The time to the first recurrence and the median time to recurrence were not significantly different between groups.[19]

Cranberry has also been shown useful in male urinary tract conditions. Half of 42 men with lower urinary tract symptoms from benign prostate disease (nonbacterial prostatitis, elevated PSA, and negative prostate biopsy) were given 1.5 grams per day of encapsulated dried cranberry powder for 6 months. In contrast to the 21 controls, the men receiving the cranberry powder showed significant improvements in urinary symptom scores including flow rate, total volume, and post-void residual urine volume, along with lower Prostate Specific Antigen (PSA) levels. In addition, the International Prostate Symptom score and quality of life were also improved significantly in the group receiving cranberry.[20] The whole berry powder appears to have more activities than simply preventing bacterial adhesion to the bladder mucosa, which was not a factor addressed in this study.

> The men receiving the cranberry powder showed significant improvements in urinary symptom scores including flow rate, total volume, and post-void residual urine volume, along with lower Prostate Specific Antigen (PSA) levels.[20]

When 12 healthy men were given 330 ml of cranberry juice to detect its effect on pH over a day, a significant acidification of the urine took place. Also, uric acid and oxalic acid content of the urine were significantly increased, while brushite and struvite urinary levels tended toward a decrease. Cranberry juice was considered a possible means for treating brushite and struvite stones.[21] In another study with 12 normal subjects and 12 calcium oxalate stone formers, consuming 1 liter of juice daily for 7 days was compared to de-ionized water effects on urine and blood chemistry. Again, urinary oxalate was significantly increased by the cranberry, while urinary pH and brushite decreased significantly. However, in this study urinary uric acid also decreased significantly, as did serum uric acid.[22]

PREVENTING BACTERIAL ADHESION

IN HUMANS

⊗⌡In a randomized, controlled, double-blind, multicentric study 295 asymptomatic children of ages 6-16 years tested positive for *Helicobacter pylori* by the C-urea breath test. Equivalent groups were given cranberry juice with the probiotic *Lactobacillus johnsonii* that was either live or heat-killed and compared with groups given placebo juice combined with the live or killed bacteria. Of the 271 that completed treatment (8.1% dropout), *H. pylori* eradication was shown to be 22.9% for cranberry/live probiotic, 16.9% cranberry/dead probiotic, 14.9% placebo/live probiotic, and 1.5% for placebo/dead probiotic. Compared to the placebo/dead probiotic group, the eradication was significant for the other 3 groups, but differences between these 3 groups were not significant.[23]⌡⊗

IN VITRO

Cranberry juice dose-dependently prevents adhesion of pathogenic *E. coli* to urinary tract mucosal tissue exposed to the urine following juice consumption, compared to exposure to urine after receiving a placebo, in a randomized crossover study with 20 subjects.[24] In an *in vitro* study of 3 commercial extracts standardized to proanthocyanidins against bacteria associated with biofilm production on urinary catheters, the inhibition of growth and biofilm production was observed at minimum concentrations ranging from 0.01-5 mg/ml for Gram-positive *Staphylococcus* spp. (including *S. epidermidis, S. aureus,* methycillin-resistant *S. aureus* [MRSA], and *S. saprophyticus*), but not for the Gram-negative *E. coli*. Also, the extracts did not eradicate established biofilms *in vitro*.[25]

The potential benefits of cranberry are not limited to the urinary tract. The anti-adhesion effect also inhibits attachment to human mucosal cells by *Helicobacter pylori*, the bacteria responsible for most gastric and duodenal ulcers and potentially leading to gastric cancer. This has been shown in a randomized, double-blind study with 189 adults with *H. pylori* infection given 250 ml of cranberry juice or placebo twice daily for 90 days. After 35 and 90 days, 14.4% of the cranberry group were negative for *H. pylori* based on urea breath test, compared to 5.4% of the placebo group.[26]

Similarly, the effects of cranberry polyphenols on *Porphyromonas gingivalis*, the main agent involved in chronic periodontitis, include reduced adhesion and formation of biofilm, along with similar effects on other species including *Treponema denticola* and *Tannerella forsythia*.[27] A cranberry fraction also inhibits adhesion of *Streptococci* and *Actinomyces* to tooth surfaces and so may help prevent cavities when taken in liquid form.[1] Cranberry juice and its 65% proanthocyanidin fraction inhibit biofilm formation and organic acid production by *Streptococcus mutans* and *S. sobrinus*. They also inhibit the adhesion of these and other streptococcal cariogenic bacteria which may further help reduce dental cavities. In addition, they decreased production of proteolytic enzymes involved in destroying the extracellular periodontal matrix.[27] The juice fraction in low concentration also reduced the metabolic activity of *S. gordonii* in biofilm may likewise benefit oral health.[28]

A 2012 review article on cranberries *in vitro* studies on bacterial anti-adhesion activity showed all 7 studies found anti-adhesion effects, 6 of 7 found the effect dose-dependent, and 5 of the 7 used post-cranberry consumption urine as the tested agent. Besides *E. coli*, other species for which mucosal adherence was inhibited by cranberry extracts include *Proteus* spp., *Pseudomonas aeruginosa*, *Enterococcus faecalis*, *Staph. aureus*, *Salmonella typhimurium*, and *Klebsiella pneumoniae*.[29] As for antimicrobial activity, results in testing 50 mcL of 4 cranberry cultivar ethanolic extracts against 10 Gram-positive and -negative species and 8 yeast found that Gram-positive *Micrococcus luteus* and *Bacillus cereus* were the most sensitive and Gram-negative *E. coli* was the least sensitive. Moderate activity was shown with some pathogenic species including *Enterococcus faecalis*, *Listeria monocytogenes*, *Salmonella typhimurium* and *Staphylococcus aureus*. The positive control combination of 30 mcg ceftazidime with 10 mcg clavulanic acid was more effective than cranberry against all bacteria except *B. cereus*. The yeast were not inhibited by the cranberry extracts.[7]

IMMUNE EFFECTS

IN HUMANS

A randomized, placebo-controlled, double-blind study used 450 ml of cranberry beverage made from juice-derived powdered cranberry fraction high in proanthocyanidins that was given to 22 healthy adults daily for 10 weeks, and the incidence and symptoms of colds and flu was compared with 23 receiving a placebo beverage. While the cranberry preparation did not affect the incidence of viral respiratory infections, the total symptoms from these infections were significantly less than for the placebo group. When peripheral blood mononuclear cells from the cranberry group were cultured *ex vivo* with phytohemagglutinin, the cell proliferation was about 5 times greater than for the placebo group. In particular, the $\gamma\delta$-T cells located in the epithelium as a first-line defense were signicantly increased.[30]

EFFECTS ON CARDIOVASCULAR DISEASE RISK FACTORS

IN HUMANS

In spite of diminished antioxidant content in the juice, consumption of cranberry juice cocktail in 30 obese men using increasing amounts of 125, 250 and 500 ml/day over three 4-week periods led to a significant increases in high-density lipoprotein (HDL) after the last two periods.[31] In this same group, matrix metalloproteinase-9, implicated in cardiovascular risk, was significantly reduced in the plasma after 12 weeks in association with significant reductions in nitrites/nitrates and systolic blood pressure.[32] In 30 healthy men of an average age of 51 years on the same dosage schedule, oxidized low-density lipoprotein (LDL), intercellular adhesion molecule-1, and vascular cell adhesion molecule-1 were all significantly decreased.[33]

Treated patients, 16 men and 14 women with type 2 diabetes, taking oral hypoglycemic medications were randomized to receive 500 mg capsules of cranberry extract or placebo 3 times daily after meals for 12 weeks. The cranberry extract group, while showing a neutral effect on glycemic control, had significantly lower total cholesterol and LDL-cholesterol than the placebo group.[34] In men with type 2 diabetes, high apoB and low apoA-1 are better predictors of high risk of cardiovascular disease than high non-HDL and low HDL, respectively. When 58 men with diabetes type 2 were given either a cup (240 ml) of cranberry juice or placebo daily for 12 weeks, those consuming the juice had significantly lower apoB and significantly higher apoA-1 than baseline values and placebo group values. Also, the fasting serum glucose was significantly lower and paraoxoanase-1, an HDL-associated enzyme, was significantly higher in the cranberry juice group than the baseline and placebo group values, as well.[35]

In coronary heart disease patients, 14 were given 480 ml double-strength cranberry juice in a single dose and showed improved brachial artery flow-mediated dilation after 4 hours in an uncontrolled acute pilot study. In 44 coronary artery disease patients given the same dose daily for 4 weeks in a randomized, placebo-controlled crossover design, the average carotid-femoral pulse wave velocity that indicated central aortic stiffness was decreased by the cranberry juice, a significant difference from the increase found with placebo, but flow-mediated dilation did not change.[36]

When 500 ml of cranberry juice cocktail (27% juice) or placebo was given daily for 4 weeks to 35 abdominally obese men, there was no significant difference in the augmentation index, a measure of arterial stiffness, between the juice and placebo groups. However, in those men with metabolic syndrome who drank the juice cocktail, the resting augmentation index values were significantly lower and the response to salbutamol and glyceryl trinitrate was significantly greater than for the men without metabolic syndrome.[37]

In 16-20 healthy subjects taking 1200 mg of dried cranberry juice daily for 4-8 weeks, the serum levels of advanced oxidation protein products was significantly decreased compared to baseline or levels of 23 taking placebo or 18-19 taking only 400 mg dried juice daily, indicating a protection against oxidative stress.[5] However, another study that gave 750 ml/day of cranberry juice for only two weeks to 20 healthy women of ages 18-40 years found no changes in LDL, HDL, or plasma antioxidant potential.[38]

In 56 individuals with metabolic syndrome, the 20 given 700 ml of low-calorie juice daily for 60 days had significant increases in serum folic acid and significant decreases in serum homocysteine, compared to baseline values. There was also significant increases in serum adiponectin and significant decreases in lipoperoxidation and protein oxidation, compared to both baseline and the control group. Groups were matched by sex, age, and ethnicity.[39] When 31 women with metabolic syndrome were randomized, 15 were given 480 ml (2 cups) daily of low calorie cranberry juice for 8 weeks and compared to a 16 given a placebo control in a double-blind manner. Compared to placebo, the juice significantly increased plasma antioxidant capacity and decreased oxidized LDL and malondialdehyde, a marker for lipoperoxidation. No significant changes were noted in glucose, lipid profiles, blood pressure, C-reactive protein, or IL-6 with this low-calorie cranberry juice.[40]

Compared to low-calorie juice and water, normal-calorie cranberry juice led to significant elevation of blood glucose after 30 minutes, but the difference was no longer significant after 180 minutes. Plasma insulin was significantly higher after 60 minutes but not after 120 minutes. Blood pressure and heart rate were unchanged.[41] Similarly, in 13 patients with type 2 diabetes the plasma glucose peak at 30 minutes was 7.0 mmol/L for 55 grams of raw cranberries, compared to 9.6 mmol/L for 40 grams sweetened dried cranberries. The plasma insulin peak for the sweetened was 157 pmol/mL at 60 minutes, whereas for the raw it was only 61 pmol/mL at 30 minutes.[42] Six capsules daily of juice powder for 6 weeks was shown to not raise fasting glucose or glycosylated hemoglobin, while after 12 weeks insulin levels were lowered, compared to placebo.[2]

In Animals

In studies of rats fed high fructose diets, the addition of freeze-dried cranberry powder at 3.3 or 6.6 grams/kg led to normalization to control values of the glucose area-under-curve following an oral glucose tolerance test, as well as improving models of insulin resistance and beta-cell function. Increases in plasma triglycerides and kidney weight due to high fructose were prevented by cranberry powder.[43]

Rats fed an atherogenic diet with or without 5% freeze-dried cranberry powder for 6 weeks had higher HDL-cholesterol than normal controls or those fed the atherogenic diet.[44,45] Average serum levels of inflammatory markers C-reactive protein and IL-1beta were significantly lower in the cranberry group than the atherogenic diet-only group. Nitric oxide and anti-inflammatory IL-10 were higher by 88% and 29%, respectively, in the cranberry group over atherogenic controls.[44] The freeze-dried cranberry powder also significantly protected against oxidation of lipids and proteins, based on other markers.[45]

Cranberry flavonoids were shown to ameliorate insulin resistance and improve plasma lipids in obese mice due to mediation of the adiponectin-AMPK pathway, whereas in normal mice these flavonoids reduced plasma cholesterol by downregulation of hepatic cholesterol synthesis.[46] Animal studies with juice powder also found a reduction of low density lipoprotein (LDL) oxidation *ex vivo* and lowering LDL levels *in vivo*.[1,2] Cardiovascular health is further promoted by reduced platelet aggregation and vasodilation, as shown in animals given cranberry juice.[2]

CANCER RESEARCH

IN HUMANS

Consumption of cranberry juice has resulted in the elevation of urinary salicylate concentrations in women who were not using aspirin or other salicylate drugs. After taking 750 ml/day for one week, salicylic acid and it metabolite, salicyluric acid, were markedly elevated in the urine, and after two weeks salicylic acid was significantly increased in the plasma. The anti-inflammatory effects of this compound may be associated in part with lowering the risk of colon cancer following consumption of fruit and vegetables.[47]

IN ANIMALS

A freeze-dried acidified methanolic fraction was made from the cranberry presscake after juice extraction. When tested against a human tumor line *in vivo*, the presscake flavonoid fraction and a whole cranberry water extract rich in PACs were injected intraperitoneally in mice. Glioblastoma multiforme tumors were significantly reduced in size by both extracts after 10 injected over 21-24 days, compared to controls, and took significantly longer to reach a series of specified sizes. The PAC extract likewise significantly inhibited the grown of colon carcinoma and prostate cancer DU145 tumor explants for which it was used, arresting growth in the G1 cell cycle phase.[48] The presscake fraction activity demonstrates the potency of compounds left behind after juice extraction, especially ursolic acid. However, results from injecting extracts cannot be extrapolated to oral dosing, due to reduced bioavailability with oral consumption.

Diets supplemented with 0.05%, 0.1%, or 0.25% ursolic acid all reduced injected mammary tumor cell growth in mice, with the 0.1% (about 106 mg/kg daily) being most effective at preventing palpable tumor growth and decreasing tumor size.[49] Even with the loss of unextracted material, cranberry juice concentrate was still shown to reduce the number of urinary bladder cancers 38% compared to placebo when given in a dose of 1.0 ml by gavage (throguh tube into stomach) daily following exposure to the carcinogenic N-butyl-N-(4-hydroxybutyl)-nitrosamine. No toxicity or weight loss ensued. Quercetin and its methylated derivative were detected in the urine.[50]

IN VITRO

The antiproliferative effect against human cancer cell lines was investigated for a total cranberry extract rich in organic acids (30.0%), total polyphenols (10.6%), PACs (5.5%), and anthocyanins (1.2%). The total extract was compared with the separated fractions for activity against human oral, colon, and prostate cancer cell lines. The most active against all cell lines was the total polyphenolic fraction. The total cranberry extract was more active than the other fractions against oral and colon cancer cell lines, while the total extract and all fractions had greater than 50% antiproliferative activity against prostate cancer cells.[51] Though exposure of colon and prostate cells *in vivo* to all of the components of the total extract or its fractions is impractical, oral tissue has immediate exposure to the entire complement of components.

More pertinent for oral dosing of liquid cranberry prepartions is its effect on oral cancer, especially the most common type, squamous cell carcinoma. In 2 well-characterized tissue cultures cranberry extract with 95% PACs, including 80-90% oligomeric PACs, dose-dependently inhibited proliferation of oral squamous cell carcinoma, as well as up-regulating caspase-2 and -8, key regulators of apoptosis. These effects were similar to those shown with grape seed extract that is also high in PACs.[52] Along with grapes and other *Vaccinium* species, cranberry is also relatively high in the antioxidant stilbene compound resveratrol that has been shown to possess cancer chemopreventive properties *in vitro*.[53]

The situation is similar for the esophagus. Esophageal adeno-carcinoma and its precursor, Barret's esophagus, are increasing rapidly over the past several decades. A proanthocyanidin-rich extract of cranberries was tested against human esophageal adenocarcinoma cells *in vitro*. The extract induced cell cycle arrest at G1 and resulted in significant apoptosis. The extract modulates cell cycle regulation, aberrant proliferation and apoptosis, all of which are altered during progession to esophageal adenocarcinoma.[54] The PAC-rich extract's demonstrated ability to modify microRNA profiles in esophageal adenocarcinoma and Barrett's esophagus is in part responsible for its cancer inhibitory potential.[55]

Another illustration of how much activity of the berry is left behind after extracting the juice, the proliferation of 8 different tumor cell lines has been shown to be inhibited by a freeze-dried acidified methanolic fraction made from the cranberry presscake after juice extraction. This fraction contained flavonols, anthocyanins, flavan-3-ols, and PACs. The minimum concentrations of this fraction that inhibited 50% of the growth (IC_{50}) for androgen receptor-negative prostate carcinoma cells (LNCaP line) was only 10 mcg/ml, while for lung cancer cells (DMS114 line) it was 21 mcg/ml. The effect was concentration dependent and continued for at least 4 days after the extract was withdrawn in an estrogen-negative breast cancer line.[56]

Similarly, a 100:1 (fresh wt.:extract) freeze-dried whole cranberry methanol and acetone extract was shown at 25 and 50 mcg/ml to significantly reduce viability of the same prostate cancer cell line (DU145) when treated for only 6 hours. This was accompanied at 50 mcg/ml by significantly decreased expression of cell cycle related proteins CDK4, cyclins A, B1, D1, and E.[56] Ursolic acid and its esters, highest in products prepared with whole fruit, inhibited DU145 tumor cell growth at micromolar concentration, due in part to inhibition of matrix metalloproteinase-2 and -9 activity.[6]

Doubling quinone reductase activity was achieved by cranberry ethyl acetate fraction at 43.7 mcg tannic acid equivalents (TAE). Cranberry crude methanolic extract at 7.0 mcg TAE and the polymeric proanthocyanidin fraction at 6.0 mcg TAE inhibited by 50% the ornithine decarboxylase activity induced by the tumor promoter phorbol 12-myristate 13-acetate.[58]

It is clear that cranberry has shown potential for inhibiting cancer development and growth preclinically, but more *in vivo* research on cranberry administered orally or by gavage as a means of chemoprevention of cancer is needed before conclusive evidence is available.[59] In addition, cranberry and blueberry have many similar compounds and activities in modulating mechanisms and markers of cancer and cardiovascular disease. The similarities are accompanied by distinctive differences as well.[60]

CRANBERRY CULTIVATION AREA, PESTICIDES, AND CANCER RISK

One concern about cranberries has to do with the use of pesticides in the process of cultivation and the subsequent risk of developing cancer of those who live near cranberry bogs. Eight types of cancer were assesed in a case-control study that looked at cases diagnosed in the Cape Cod area of Massachusetts from 1983 to 1986. The incidence of leukemia and cancers of the lung, breast, colon/rectum, bladder, kidney, pancreas, and brain were compared between those living in proximity to cranberry bogs and control subjects randomly selected from telephone subscribers, Medicare beneficiaries, and deceased subjects. There was no increased risk associated with having ever lived within 2600 ft of a cranberry bog for 7 of the cancers, but brain cancer risk was 2-fold greater overall, and 6.7-fold greater for astrocytoma.[61]

Since many pesticides mimic estrogen, a further population-based case-control study was undertaken with 1,165 women diagnosed with breast cancer from 1988-1995 who were residents of Cape Cod. Comparisons were made to 1,006 controls. A modest increase in breast cancer risk was associated with the aerial application on cranberry bogs of persistent pesticides.[62] The need for pesticide use for the gypsy moth increased with selection for cultivars that have increased yields and fruit quality traits but lower concentrations of self-defensive phytochemicals.[63]

CRANBERRY IN PREGNANCY

Women suffer from UTIs more frequently in pregnancy, and a survey of 400 postpartem women found that, though cranberry was one of the most commonly used "herbs" during pregnancy, no adverse events were associated with its regular consumption.[64] The Norwegian Mother and Child Cohort Study of 68,522 pregnant women found that 919 had used cranberry. Use in pregnancy was not associated with any increased risk of neonatal death or stillbirth, or low birth weight, preterm birth, small for gestational age, Apgar score of <7, neonatal infections, or vaginal bleeding in early pregnancy. Maternal vaginal bleeding pregnancy after week 17 of gestation was associated with cranberry use in late pregnancy, but not severe bleeding. Of the 554 cases of UTIs in which cranberry was ingested, 300 did not employ antibiotics. Cranberry has not been shown to be effective in treatment of UTIs. UTIs with exposure to cranberry but without antibiotic treatment had increased odds ratios for stillbirth/neonatal death, small for gestational age, and neonatal infections, so cranberry should not be relied upon for treating UTIs in pregnancy.[65]

> Though cranberry was one of the most commonly used "herbs" during pregnancy, no adverse events were associated with its regular consumption.[64]

WARFARIN INTERACTION RISK

Contrary to case reports suggesting cranberry juice may inhibit S-warfarin metabolism, a human study with 10 healthy subjects taking 200 ml of the juice or water 3 times daily for 10 days found the juice has no significant effect on S-warfarin metabolic enzymes CYP2C9 or

CYP3A, nor did it change warfarin's anticoagulant effect.[66] This was confirmed with 30 patients on stable warfarin anticoagulation dosage who were randomized to consume 240 ml of cranberry juice or water once daily for 2 weeks. The average concentrations of plasma R- and S-warfarin did not differ between groups, and 4 patients in both groups showed slightly elevated INRs.[67]

> The juice has no significant effect on S-warfarin metabolic enzymes CYP2C9 or CYP3A, nor did it change warfarin's anticoagulant effect.[66]

CRANBERRY EXTRACTS FOR RADIATION CYSTITIS

In a study with 370 patients treated with radiation for prostate cancer, for 6-7 weeks 184 of the men daily received 200 mg of enteric-coated cranberry extract standardized to 30% PACs. Only 8.7% of patients on cranberry had lower urinary tract infections, significantly lower than the 24.2% on placebo. In addition, cranberry extract significantly reduced dysuria, nocturia, and urinary urgency and frequency, compared to placebo, indicating a general protective effect.[68]

In a randomized, placebo-controlled, double-blind study with 40 men with prostate cancer treated by radiation for 9-10 weeks, half received a capsule of cranberry extract with 72 mg of PACs daily during treatment plus 2 weeks afterward. Those taking the cranberry extract had a lower incidence of radiation cystitis (65% vs. 90%) and significantly less pain/burning.[69]

> Those taking the cranberry extract had a lower incidence of radiation cystitis (65% vs. 90%) and significantly less pain/burning.[69]

SUMMARY

The usefulness of cranberry juice as a means of preventing urinary tract infections among women is well recognized, due primarily to its anti-adhesion effect on *E. coli* and/or other pathogenic bacteria, and its use in early pregnancy for this purpose may be effective and appears to be safe. However, it is not advisable for use as a treatment for bladder infections, especially in late pregnancy. Whole cranberry powder and powdered extract are also effective without the need for added sweeteners. While the use of whole cranberry powder for urinary symptoms in benign prostatic conditions in men may be advantageous, its benefits for bladder symptoms from treating prostate cancer with radiation are becoming more evident.

Cranberry products have also been found to provide potential usefulness as chemopreventive agents. The most compelling *in vivo* studies with cranberry freeze-dried powder or human research using extracts and juice point to the benefits that can be derived for helping to prevent and reduce cardiovascular disease risk markers. This is particularly true for patients who are obese and/or have type 2 diabetes or metabolic syndrome. A disadvantage of cranberry products that have added sugar(s) is the increase in plasma glucose, but when considering the potential benefits, it is clear that cranberries are not only good for Thanksgiving.

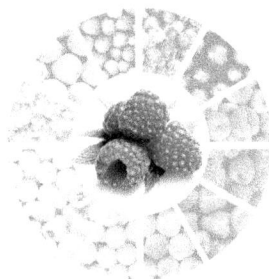

F O U R

ROSE FAMILY *RUBUS* AND *ARONIA* BERRIES

AMONG NATIVE AMERICAN BLACKBERRIES AND RASPBERRIES OF THE ROSACEAE (ROSE) FAMILY RUBUS GENUS, THE BLACK RASPBERRY IS NOTEWORTHY FOR ITS SIZE AND VALUE. AS A REPRESENTATIVE OF THIS DIVERSE GENUS OF FOOD PLANTS, BLACK RASPBERRY WILL BE DISCUSSED FOR ITS SEEMINGLY UNIQUE CONTRIBUTION FOR MAINTAINING HEALTH BY HELPING TO REDUCE THE DEVELOPMENT OF ALIMENTARY TRACT CANCERS. WITHIN THE ARONIA GENUS OF THE SAME FAMILY, THE BLACK CHOKEBERRY IS AN ESPECIALLY RICH SOURCE OF VALUABLE POLYPHENOLIC ANTIOXIDANTS, PROVIDING ONE OF THE HIGHEST CONTENTS OF ANTHOCYANINS AND PROCYANIDINS AND GREATEST ANTIOXIDANT VALUES OF ALL PLANTS MEASURED TO DATE.

The most popular berry of the Rose family is undoubtedly the strawberry, first cultivated as the woodland European species (*Fragaria vesca*) in the early 17th century, but now usually sold commercially as the hybrid of North and South American species (*Fragaria × ananassa*). Like the strawberry, other berry plants of the Rose family are not of the luxuriant floral variety as the beautiful *Rosa* species for which the family is named, but may like the *Rubus* species harbor thorns on the stems. Some of the familiar commercial *Rubus* species originally from Europe are now grown in America, including red raspberry (*R.

idaeus), European bramble or blackberry (*R. fruticosus*) and evergreen blackberry (*E. lanciniatus*).

Many species of the *Rubus* genus are native to North America. Among these, blackberries are widespread but regional, and most occur only in the wild such as Pacific blackberry (*R. vitifolius* syn. *R. ursinus*). The most familiar American blackberry is *R. villosus* in the northeastern and central United States. Blackberries have thorny stems, known as canes, that bear leaves the first year and fruit the second year, after which they die. Currently, the American blackberry cultivars are grown from leafy stem cuttings or root cuttings after being hybridized from many wild species. The major areas of production are in the Pacific Northwest, Michigan, and Arkansas.

The major difference between raspberries and blackberries is that when a raspberry is picked ripe, it has a hollow center since the torus (receptacle of the inflorescence) remains on the cane. This gives the berry a hollow appearance on the stem end, so that it resembles a cap. Blackberries, in contrast to raspberries, retain the torus which is consumed as part of the berry. Several wild species of raspberries are native to North America such as the Western blackcap or blue raspberry (*R. leucodermis*) in the Pacific Northwest. American red raspberry (*R. strigosus*) in the Northeast is known for both its fruit and its leaf used in herbal teas. Thimbleberry (*R. parviflorus*) and salmonberry (R. *spectabilis*) that grow wild near the Pacific coast share the fruit structure of raspberries.

The black raspberry (*Rubus occidentalis*), though increasing in commercial cultivar development, is not as widespread in the wild nor as broadly cultivated as blackberries. As with other *Rubus* species, black raspberry shares with strawberries a high content of the anticarcinogenic ellagic acid, but its concentration in the small hard seeds normally reduces the bioavailability. Though there have not been extensive human studies on black raspberry's effects, there has been significant preclinical research on the powdered freeze-dried fruit and its major components. This is especially true regarding the prevention of cancers of the mouth, esophagus, and gastrointestinal tract.

Aronia species of the Rose family are deciduous understory shrubs native to eastern North America including Canada. Commonly known as chokeberries due to the astringency of the berries, the two main species are the black chokeberry (*Aronia melanocarpa*) and the red chokeberry (*A. arbutifolia*). The commercial development of these continues to grow; the sweeter red berries persist into winter, while black chokeberries do not. A purported natural hybrid of these is the purple chokeberry (*A. prunifolia*), considered by some as a separate species as it grows in regions where neither parent species occurs.

The much darker black chokeberry is particularly high in antioxidant anthocyanins and the astringent procyanidins. American black chokeberries were introduced to eastern Europe in the 20th century and are now grown extensively in northeastern Europe. These plants have at times been grouped with the genus *Photinia*, but recent molecular studies decidedly refute a close relationship. Chokeberries should not be mistaken with the chokecherry (*Prunus virginiana*).

Research data on different black raspberry cultivars is emphasized in cases of comparative phytochemical content studies between them. As noted below, much of the preclinical research utilizes the Ohio-grown black raspberry Jewel cultivar, but this and other cultivars vary in content depending on location and maturity. In addition, the specific cultivars utilized may not be noted by some researchers, so, in general, little attempt has been made to compare the pharmacological differences. The three different chokeberry species are compared phytochemically, but otherwise the research specifically involves black chokeberry, referred to throughout the discussion simply as chokeberry.

Black Raspberry

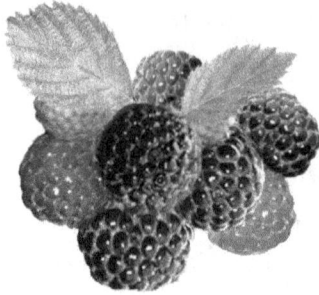

THE CONSISTENT EFFECT OF FREEZE-DRIED BLACK RASPBERRIES IN VIVO HAS BEEN TO REDUCE THE DEVELOPMENT OF CANCER FROM PRECANCEROUS CONDITIONS OR INDUCED BY CARCINOGENIC SUBSTANCES. ANTHOCYANINS OF BLACK RASPBERRY SUCH AS CYANIDIN-3-RUTINOSIDE ARE LIMITED BY THEIR POOR ABSORPTION, LEADING TO MORE LOCAL EFFECTS IN REDUCING CANCER DEVELOPMENT ALONG THE ALIMENTARY TRACT FROM THE MOUTH TO THE RECTUM. ITS SYSTEMIC PROTECTION IS MORE LIKELY DUE TO ELLAGIC ACID, MADE MORE AVAILABLE THROUGH POWDERING THE FREEZE-DRIED BERRY WITH ITS SEEDS. HOWEVER, NO SINGLE COMPONENT OR EXTRACT FRACTION HAS BEEN ABLE TO DUPLICATE THE EFFICACY OF THE WHOLE BERRY. MUCH OF THE CHEMOPREVENTIVE RESEARCH ON BLACK RASPBERRIES IS WITH ORAL CONSUMPTION OF THE FREEZE-DRIED BERRIES.

Often referred to as black caps, black raspberries (*Rubus occidentalis*) are native to the eastern United States, but most are now grown commercially in western Oregon. There are a number of varieties that differ in production and climactic preferences. Much research has been done with the Jewel variety grown in Ohio, while the Munger cultivar is the most common variety grown in Oregon. Commercial yield is small compared to other species of berries, and replanting is required every 3-4 years, making black raspberries more expensive than many other berries.[1]

Though sharing the same *Rubus* genus as other caneberries such as red raspberry and blackberry, the anthocyanin constituent profile and content, bioactivity, and the flavor of black raspberry are distinctive from the others. Specifically, black raspberries have the highest oxygen radical absorbance capacity (ORAC) value of the caneberries, 3 times that of red raspberries and blackberries, in association with twice the amount of ellagic acid and total phenolics of either of these, and 6.5 to 9 times the anthocyanin content, respectively, along with different major anthocyanins.[2]

Black raspberries have the highest oxygen radical absorbance capacity (ORAC) value of the caneberries.[2]

Phenolic Content of Berries and Seeds

Freeze-dried black raspberries yield large amounts of both anthocyanins and ellagic acid. The primary anthocyanidins in *R. occidentalis* Jewel cultivar from 4 commercial growers in Ohio as shown in one study were cyanidin-3-rutinoside (24-40%) and cyanidin-3-xylosylrutinoside (49-58%).[3] In another study, an Ohio Jewel variety provided 60% cyanidin-3-rutinoside and 29% cyanidin-3-xylosylrutinoside.[4] In Jewel cultivar berries grown in Oregon, these two anthocyanins were present in almost equal amounts, whereas the Munger cultivar berries had much higher cyanidin-3-rutinoside content than cyanidin-3-xylosylrutinoside.[1] Black raspberries are obviously a rich source of both of these potent antioxidant anthocyanins, along with lesser amounts of cyanidin-3-glucoside, cyanidin-3-sambubioside, pelargonidin-3-rutinoside, and traces of other anthocynanins.[1,3,4]

Ellagitannins are another major class of bioactive polyphenols in black raspberries. Like most *Rubus* caneberries, about half of the total ellagic acid in these berries is in the form of ellagitannins, while the other half is free ellagic acid.[2] Besides containing large amounts of anthocyanins and ellagic acid, freeze-dried blackberries, washed and frozen within 1-4 hours of picking, yield significant amounts of beta-sitosterol, ferulic acid, calcium, and fiber.[4,5] Comparing component concentrations in freeze-dried powder from harvests in 1997, 2001, and 2006, beta-sitosterol ranged from 80-110 mg/100 g, ferulic acid from 5-47 mg/100 g, and calcium from 175-215 mg/100 g.[6]

By freeze-drying and powdering black raspberries, the nutrient content of the seeds is released to an extent that is not possible with ordinary consumption of fresh or frozen black raspberries, or any of the caneberries. One component that is especially high in black raspberry seeds compared to the pulp is ellagic acid. For example, in a sample of ripe Ohio Jewel black raspberries in 1996, the ellagic acid content of the seeds was twice as much as the pulp, while in 1997 it was 14 times as much.[7] (Similar ranges were seen with red raspberries and blackberries, with the seeds always proportionally containing much higher quantities of ellagic acid.[7,8])

> One component that is especially high in black raspberry seeds compared to the pulp is ellagic acid.[7]

While the total phenolic content of the seeds and ORAC value were lower than those for the whole dried black raspberry fruit, the seed powder still inhibited colon cancer cells dose-dependently *in vitro*.[9] The total phenolic content and free radical scavenging capacity of the seed meal was 300 times greater than that of the oil isolated from the seeds which contained 35% alpha-linolenic acid and 55-58% linoleic acid.[10]

BIOAVAILABILITY OF BLACK RASPBERRY ANTHOCYANINS AND ELLAGIC ACID

IN HUMANS

In a study with 11 subjects (1 woman), 45 grams of freeze-dried black raspberries were consumed daily for 7 days. The maximum blood concentrations of ellagic acid and the 4 major cyanidin anthocyanins occurred 1 to 2 hours after black raspberry consumption, while highest content in the urine was found in the first 4 hours after eating the berries. Less than 1% of these constituents were found in the urine. These finding did not change from day 1 to day 7. The berries were well-tolerated.[11]

A similar study with 10 men using 45 grams daily of freeze-dried black raspberries (providing about 2.7 grams of anthocyanins per day) for a week again showed that they were well tolerated. However, in this study most of the anthocyanins excreted in the urine in the first 12 hours appeared 4-8 hours after consumption. It was also noted that even though cyanidin 3-xylosylrutinoside accounted for about 26% of the total anthocyanins in the berries, it was present in the urine in much higher concentrations than cyanidin 3-rutinoside that provided about 60% of the berry anthocyanins. Small amounts of metabolites in the urine were methylated derivatives of the anthocyanins.[12]

Protocatechuic acid, a major black raspberry anthocyanin metabolite generated by microbial metabolism, has antioxidant and anti-carcinogenic activities. In 5 prostate cancer patients consuming 60 grams of freeze-dried black raspberry powder daily for 20 days, protocatechuic acid was detectable in all 5 with a mean plsma concentration of 3.9 ng/ml.[13]

> Protocatechuic acid, a major black raspberry anthocyanin metabolite generated by microbial metabolism, has antioxidant and anti-carcinogenic activities.[13]

In Animals

In a study with 30 rats, the aqueous fraction of a 70% acetonic extract of freeze-dried black raspberries was itself freeze-dried and was administered by stomach tube. The animals were sacrificed after 0.5, 1, 2, and 3 hours, and the anthocyanin content in the stomach and intestine were analyzed. The anthocyanin glycosides remained stable in the stomach. Uptake in the small intestine tissue peaked at 120 minutes, and the mucosal tissue content reached 7.5% of the amount of anthocyanins consumed. Decrease of cyanidin 3-glucoside in the small intestine lumen was likely due to bacterial beta-glucosidase activity. Urinary profiles reflected the gastrointestinal content.[14]

Freeze-dried black raspberries given to 5 weanling pigs that were sacrificed after 4 hours showed that the total anthocyanins in the small intestine and colon at that time amounted to 42% of the total, mostly in the ileum, cecum, and colon. The cyanidin glycosides were recovered at different rates, depending on the sugar moieties. The amounts recovered in the urine were consistent with the stability of the anthocyanins in the GI tract which varied according to the environment of the different segments. The more complex anthocyanins were more stable than the simpler monoglycosides. After 4 hours, the amount in the gut (42% of the total anthocyanins consumed) and its antioxidant activity (46.5% of the initial amount) indicate that the antioxidant protection provided by black raspberries for the gut epithelium is significant.[15]

Other polyphenolics in berries are often converted to smaller phenolic acids by microbes in the colon. These metabolites may contribute to the health benefits of the berries. The primary phenolic acids excreted in the urine following 5% freeze-dried black raspberry dietary intake by rats are 3-hydroxycinnamic acid, 3-hydroxybenzoic acid, and 3-hydroxyphenylpropionic acid. In contrast, major urinary phenolic acids following a diet with 5% freeze-dried blueberries were chlorogenic, ferulic, and 3,4-dihydroxycinnamic acids, while after a 5% freeze-dried cranberry diet it was 4-hydroxycinnamic acid.[16]

CANCER CELL GROWTH: POTENTIAL FOR PREVENTING OR REDUCING WITH WHOLE BERRIES OR DERIVATIVES

While whole freeze-dried black raspberries are typically used in the following human and animal cancer-prevention studies, work done on cells in the laboratory require the use of extracts or components to allow for effective exposure. This also simplifies the phytochemical content and allows better opportunity to specifically study certain compounds and their activities to help determine the mechanistic effects on cell function. This is illustrated with black raspberry derivatives used in cultures of cells from the mouth. These demonstrated *in vitro* cellular effects may be more applicable to local *in vivo* effects than many *in vitro* studies, since black raspberries come in direct contact with the oral, esophageal, or colon mucosa when consumed fresh, frozen and thawed, or freeze-dried and mixed with water.

In addition, when extracts can be applied directly to skin or mucosal surfaces, the *in vitro* results may also be pertinent. For example, in 3 lines of human cervical cancer cells (HeLa adenocarcinoma, SiHa squamous cell carcinoma, C-33A squamous cell carcinoma), a freeze-dried black raspberry ethanol extract was tested at 4 concentrations from 25 to 200 mcg/ml for 1, 3, or 5 days. Significant inhibition of cervical cancer cell growth occurred with the extract at non-toxic levels in a dose- and time-dependent manner to maximums of 54%, 52%, and 67% for the 3 cell lines, respectively. The growth inhibition continued even after a short-term withdrawal of the extract from the medium. The extract also induced apoptosis in all 3 cell lines.[17] Correspondingly, ellagic acid at 10^{-5} M has been shown to block mitosis of cervical carcinoma cells *in vitro* by G1 arrest after 48 hours, induces apoptosis in these cells, and inhibits overall cell growth after 72 hours.[18]

Oral Precancers and Cancerous Cells

In Humans

In a multicenter, placebo-controlled clinical trial with 40 patients receiving topical treatment for premalignant oral intraepithelial lesion, 22 had applied 0.5 g of a gel made with 10% freeze-dried black raspberry powder 4 times daily for 12 weeks. At the end of the trial, the lesions treated with the black raspberry gel were reduced significantly in size, histological grade, and loss of heterozygosity (LOH) events, whereas lesions treated with placebo gel had increased significantly in size.[19]

The topical application 4 times daily for 6 weeks of 0.5 grams of a bioadhesive gel with 10% freeze-dried black raspberry on premalignant oral intraepithelial neoplasia in 20 patients suppressed the genes associated with growth factor recycling, RNA processing, and inhibition of apoptosis. There were significant reductions in epithelial COX-2 proteins. Also, in a subset of patients the vascular densities in superficial connective tissues was reduced, and genes for keratinocyte differentiation were induced. Reduced proapoptotic expression and increased COX-2 are correlated with malignant transformation of these neoplasia into oral squamous cell carcinoma, suggesting potential benefits from the gel application. Histopathologic improvement was seen in 7 patients, no change in 9 patients, and disease progression in 4 patients. There were no adverse effects in the 20 patients or in 10 healthy control subjects.[20] Significant reduction in loss of heterozygosity seen at loci of tumor suppresor genes also suggests its usefulness in chemoprevention.[21]

To examine the relative bioavailability to the oral tissues of the anthocyanins when supplied as a rinse, 3 different rinse formulas were used by 10 healthy subjects, each containing 10% freeze-dried black raspberries. One used only water as vehicle, another used a suspending vehicle formula with gums and a sugar-free flavoring agent with glycerin, while the third contained the suspenion formula and flavorings along with the antimicrobial agent chlorhexidine. Tissue enzyme studies identified 7 enzymes impacting the pharmacokinetics of the anthocyanins, such as the bioactivating beta-glucosidase that releases the aglycone cyanidin.[22]

The anthocyanins and their metabolites and conjugates were present in the saliva for up to 4 hours after rinsing for 3 minutes with the 3 preparations, showing significantly better sustained levels of total anthocyanins and cyanidin-3-rutinoside than the gel used in the prior human study. The rinse with only the water had the highest anthocyanin levels over the 4 hours, but the one with the suspending and flavoring agents was the only one producing detectable protocatechuic acid in most subjects after 4 hours. The recycling of these components in the oral mucosa resembled the process that occurs in the intestines, with interpatient differences determining the retention of, and sustained exposure to, the bioactive metabolites cyanidin and protocatechuic acid that contribute to therapeutic effectiveness.[22]

The anthocyanins and their metabolites and conjugates were present in the saliva for up to 4 hours after rinsing for 3 minutes.[22]

These studies demonstrates the advantage of using the freeze-dried black raspberry powder in water, other liquids, or gels to provide exposure to the oral mucosa, especially for those who are smokers and have a higher incidence of oral neoplasia, rather than merely taking the powder in a capsule and, in so doing, bypassing the oral tissue.

In Vitro

An ethanol-extracted fraction of freeze-dried black raspberries was shown to significantly inhibit the growth of both premalignant and malignant oral epithelial cell lines without inhibiting normal epithelial cells. This same inhibitory pattern was found with the individual components ferulic acid and beta-sitosterol, neither of which was cytotoxic, unlike ellagic acid that was cytotoxic to the cell lines. The content of these 3 components in black raspberries is 166–200 mg/100g ellagic acid, and 72–89 mg/100g beta-sitosterol, and 18–21 mg/100g ferulic acid. The growth inhibition was due to inhibiting regulatory proteins of the cell cycle indifferent phases. Cell growth was blocked in the G_0/G_1 phase by beta-sitosterol in the premalignant cell line and in the G_2/M phase by beta-sitosterol in the malignant cell line and by ferulic acid in both cell lines.[23]

An ethanol extract of freeze-dried black raspberries was tested on 4 cell lines derived from human oral squamous cell carcinoma of the tongue. The extract was shown to significantly suppress cell proliferation in all cell lines without being cytotoxic at concentrations of 10 mcg/ml and above. The extract inhibited the translation and expression of vascular endothelial growth factor (VEGF) in 3 of 4 cell lines, while significantly suppressing nitric oxide synthase (NOS) activity in all 4 cell lines. VEGF and NOS elevations are associated with aggressive squamous cell carcinoma of the mouth and of the head and neck, respectively. The extract induced caspase activity in 3 of the 4 cell lines and activates the transglutamase enzyme in all cell lines, effects associated with induction of both apoptosis and terminal differentiation. The 4 main anthocyanins were all shown to be internalized in the squamous cell carcinoma cells when lysed.[24]

ESOPHAGEAL CARCINOGENESIS

IN HUMANS

Barrett's esophagus is a premalignant condition in which normal stratified squamous epithelium changes to metaplastic columnar epithelium that includes goblet cells, associated with a 30-40% increased risk of esophageal adenocarcinoma. Based upon success in animal models, a 6-month chemopreventive pilot study for Barrett's esophagus using freeze-dried black raspberries looked at daily administering 32 grams to females and 45 grams to males. The freeze-dried powder, in amounts chosen to approximate 1.5 or 2 cups of fresh black raspberries, approximating 5% of the daily diet, was mixed with 170 ml of water and taken in the morning.[25]

In a preliminary report of the first 10 patients (including 3 women) to complete the study, the intervention reduced significantly the overall average level of a marker of oxidative stress in the urine, 8-epi-prostaglandin $F2\alpha$, and its average individual urinary level in 6 of the 10 patients, compared to baseline. Another urinary oxidative stress marker, 8-hydroxy-2'-deoxyguanosine, was significantly reduced in 5 or the 10 subjects, but significantly raised in 4 others.[25]

IN ANIMALS

In rat tumor-prevention studies, the carcinogen N-nitrosomethyl-benzylamine (NMBA) is often injected subcutaneously 15 times over a number of weeks to induce 100% formation of squamous papilloma tumors in the esophagus by 26 weeks, the number of tumors depending on the dosage. These tumors mimic the squamous cell carcinomas in humans often induced by nitrosamines like NMBA. Black raspberry interventions have been studied as prevention when given before, during and after tumor initiation by NMBA, as anti-promotion when given immediately after NMBA initiation of carcinogenesis, and as therapeutic when given beginning a couple of weeks after established NMBA carcinogenesis.[26]

Freeze-dried black raspberries were fed to rats as 5% of the diet before, during and after exposure to the esophageal carcinogen NMBA or only after NMBA exposure. Demonstrating its preventive effects at 25 weeks, the incidence of papillomatous esophageal tumors in the black raspberry-treated animals were reduced by 21% and the tumor multiplicity by 41%, compared to the NMBA controls. The inhibition correlated with reduced formation of O^6-methylguanine (OmG) adduct in esophageal DNA. This preventive protection was shown to involve both inhibition of multiple initiation and post-initiation events in carcinogenesis, as well as down-regulation of key genes such as COX-2 and inducible nitric oxide synthase. The amount used would be equivalent to consuming 1.4-2.0 cups of fresh berries, or about 30-40 grams of freeze-dried berries, daily for humans.[5]

In another prevention trial, 5% or 10% of freeze-dried black raspberries in the diet were fed to rats for 2 weeks before a 15-week weekly exposure to NMBA and continued throughout the 30-week study. The tumor multiplicity was significantly reduced by the 2 berry doses at the end by 39% and 49%, respectively. The powder inhibited formation of the promutagenic adduct OmG by 73% and 80%, respectively, after a single exposure to NMBA. When used as an anti-promotion agent, beginning after 5 weeks of 3-times weekly NMBA, at 25 weeks the powder as 5% and 10% of the diet reduced esophageal neoplastic lesions, cellular proliferation, tumor incidence by 54% and 46%, respectively, and tumor multiplicity by 64% and 43%, respectively. These effects were only seen at the 5% dosage level at 35 weeks.[27]

In another study of post-initiation progression of carcinogenesis, rats were treated 3 times weekly for 5 weeks with NMBA, then beginning the next week 5% dietary freeze-dried black raspberries were given for 25 weeks. At 25 weeks, tumor multiplicity was significantly reduced from 3.78 tumors per rat in controls to 2.23 in those receiving the 5% berry powder in the diet. The powder group had reduced mRNA expression and protein levels of inducible nitric oxide synthase (iNOS), COX-2, and *c-Jun* in the pre-neoplastic esophageal lesions, along with lower prostaglandin E_2 levels.[28]

Using the same berry dosing protocol, VEGF expression in the esophagus was determined to analyze the effect on angiogenesis. The black raspberries significantly suppressed esophageal VEGF-C mRNA expression (upregulated in esophageal squamous cell carcinoma and in cancers of the head and neck, lung, breast, thyroid, stomach, uterus, prostate, and colon) from a 2.4-fold increase with NMBA alone to 1.1-fold with the NMBA and berry combination. This correlated with a decrease in COX-2 and iNOS. Also, the microvessel density of the esophagus was significantly decreased from 53.7 vessels/cm with NMBA to 22.6 vessels/cm with the added berries.[29]

It was found that a 1-week exposure of NMBA in rats via 3 subcutaneous injections led to 2,261 genes being dysregulated in the esophagus by 1.5-fold or greater. A diet with 5% freeze-dried black raspberries consumed for 2 weeks prior maintained the levels of expression near normal for 462 of the dysregulated genes. Of these, 53 included genes that are involved in phase I and phase II metabolism, oxidative damage, and genes that regulate apoptosis, cell cycling, and angiogenesis. Twenty were classified as cell junction, motility and adhesion genes.[30] For rats on the 5% berry diet for 3 weeks without exposure to NMBA, 12 genes were down-regulated, and 24 genes were up-regulated. Those up-regulated are associated with signaling cascades, transcription, apoptosis, metabolism, cellular matrix, and contraction. Most down-regulated genes had to do with cell regulation, metabolism, and signal transduction. Morphology was not impacted.[31]

Still another study in which rats were fed 5% freeze-dried black raspberry powder after NMBA injections showed at 35 weeks that the powder decreased the number of dysplastic lesions and the size and number of papillomas in the esophagus. The berry powder modulated expression of over 620 genes in both the preneoplastic lesions and the papillomas in this late stage of carcinogenesis. Associated with this was the altered mRNA expression of genes for cell proliferation and death, inflammation, apoptosis, and angiogenesis, as well as modulating matrix metalloproteinases and proteins involved with cell-cell adhesion.[32]

To help determine which components were contributing to the antitumorigenic effect, rats were fed diets with either 5% of the freeze-dried berries or extract fractions of the berries for 2 weeks before NMBA and throughout the duration of the study. The berries and the fractions rich in anthocyanins were effective in reducing tumorigenesis, as was an organic-insoluble residue fraction. They inhibited cell proliferation, angiogenesis, and inflammation, and induced apoptosis in papillomatous and preneoplastic esophageal tissues. The hexane extract and a sugar fraction had only traces of anthocyanins and were ineffective. Apparently, anthocyanins are major, but not the only, anti-tumorigenic components in black raspberry.[33]

> Anthocyanins are major, but not the only, anti-tumorigenic components in black raspberry.[33]

After including the free ellagic acid component in the diet for 3 weeks, the amount of OmG (a DNA adduct derived from NMBA) following injection of NMBA was significantly reduced in esophageal tissue of rats.[34] However, an alcohol/water-insoluble fraction of freeze-dried black raspberries, lacking anthocyanins but high in ellagitannins and given at 0.62 g/kg of diet given for 2 weeks before NMBA, was no more effective in reducing NMBA tumorigenesis in rat esophagi than an alcohol/water-insoluble fraction of freeze-dried blueberries given accordingly, but providing ellagitannins at only 0.01 g/kg of the diet. This suggests that complex ellagitannins may not contribute significantly to the anti-tumorigenic effect.[35]

As regards a potential therapeutic effect for esophageal tumors, when freeze-dried black raspberries were given as 5%, 10%, or 20% of the diet of rats for 7 weeks beginning 2 days after a 15-day exposure to NMBA, it had no significant effect on tumor development or on survival.[26] Also, since reflux-induced esophagitis is a strong risk factor for developing esophageal adenocarcinoma, freeze-dried black raspberry was tested in rats for potentially ameliorating the esophagitis induced in an esophagoduodenal anastomosis model. No alterations of the grade of esophagitis, increases in antioxidant enzymes, or reduction in lipid peroxidation were seen, compared with controls. This demonstrates the differences in the mechanisms of development of esophageal squamous cell carcinoma versus adenocarcinoma.[36]

In an attempt to identify the primary active component(s) of black raspberry in cancer prevention, rats given NMBA 3 times/week for 5 weeks to induce esophageal squamous cell carcinoma where then fed only a control diet or that diet supplemented with equivalent amounts of either freeze-dried black raspberry powder (6.1%), anthocyanin-enriched fraction (3.8 mcmol/g), or protocatechuic acid (500 ppm). While all 3 supplements significantly reduced the number of tumors and total tumor volume per rat compared to controls after 25 and 35 weeks, the whole black raspberry powder was significantly more effective for these parameters than the anthocyanin fraction or protocatechuic acid after 35 weeks. All 3 supplements also led to significant reductions in expression of sEH after 15 and 35 weeks and in iNOS (except for anthocyanin fraction) and COX-2 expression after 35 weeks, as well as significant up-regulation of the cytokine anti-inflammatory marker petraxin-3, compared to controls.[37] This study demonstrates the superiority of the whole black raspberry powder over the main active fraction or major active metabolite.

In Vitro

After freeze-dried black raspberries were fed as 5% or 10% of a diet to rats for 3 weeks, they were euthanized and the esophagi and livers were removed. These tissues exposed to NMBA were shown to inhibit NMBA phase I metabolism and its carcinogenic bioactivation in esophageal explant cultures (by 26% and 20%, respectively), probably by inhibiting CYP2A3, and also in liver microsomes (by 22% and 28%, respectively) taken from the rats, likely by CYP2E1 inhibition. In addition, phase II detoxification activity by glutathione-S-transferase in the liver was induced. These tissues from control rats not given the berry powder were exposed *in vitro* to an ethanol extract of the freeze-dried berries or to ellagic acid, cyanidin-3-glucoside, or cyanidin-3-rutinoside. The inhibition of NMBA metabolism in liver microsomes by these were 11% for the extract, 33% for ellagic acid, 32% for cyanidin-3-glucoside, and 47% for cyanidin-3-rutinoside.[38] In a highly tumorigenic cell line, the ethanolic extract and both anthocyanins significantly inhibited growth and induced apoptosis; the anthocyanins from the extract were taken up well by these cells, but not by a weak tumorigenic line that was unaffected.[39]

POTENTIAL EFFECTS ON COLON AND RECTAL TUMORS AND MUCOSAL OXIDATION OR INFLAMMATION

IN HUMANS

After biopsying cancerous tissue and adjacent normal tissue, 20 grams of freeze-dried black raspberry powder was given 3 times daily for 1 to 9 weeks to 6 patients with colon adenocarcinomas and 14 patients with rectal adenocarcinomas. The average patient age was 59 years; 17 were male, and 2 had metastasis. Anthocyanins were detected in both tissue types and in the urine after treatment. In those receiving an average of 4 weeks of black raspberry treatment (avg. 83 doses), but not those with an average of 2 weeks treatment (avg. 52 doses), post-treatment biopsies showed modulation in a protective direction in 4 of 5 tested tumor suppressor genes in cancerous and normal colorectal tissue via demethylation. Three of the genes were associated with the Wnt pathway and impacted biomarkers for proliferation, apoptosis, and angiogenesis. These changes were associated with decreased DNA methyltransferase I protein expression.[40] The study of anthocyanins from black raspberry demonstrated that they are responsible at least in part for the demethylation effects in colorectal cancer.[41]

Plasma and colorectal adenocarcinoma tissue collected from 24 colorectal cancer patients, before and after consuming 60 grams of freeze-dried black raspberry powder daily for 1-9 weeks, showed a significant decrease in interleukin (IL)-8 and a significant increase in granulocyte macrophage colony stimulating factor in the plasma. This correlated with beneficial changes in colorectal tissue markers for apoptosis and cell proliferation in the same time frame.[42]

When 28 colorectal cancer patients consumed 60 grams per day of freeze-dried black raspberry powder for 1 to 9 weeks, most alterations were with lipids. Plasma samples showed a decrease in monosaturated fatty acid eicosenoate and the polyunsaturated fatty acids linoleate and arachindonate and secondary bile acids like glycodeoxycholate. The reduction in fatty acids may be associated with inhibition of phospholipase A, elongase, or saturase enzymes, while bile acid metabolism alteration is likely due to changes in colonic microflora.

Changes in bile acid metabolism can affect lipid absorption and metabolism.[43]

IN ANIMALS

Rats with azoxymethane-induced aberrant crypt foci and colon tumors were given diets with 2.5%, 5%, or 10% freeze-dried black raspberries. After 33 weeks those receiving the berry powder had significantly less total tumors (42%, 45%, and 71%, respectively) and less adenocarcinoma multiplicity (28%, 35%, and 80%, respectively) than control rats, dose-dependently. Urinary levels of the DNA adduct 8-hydroxy-2'-deoxyguanosine, a marker of oxidative stress, were significantly reduced by 73-83% dose-dependently, as well.[44]

Feeding the freeze-dried berries for 12 weeks to mice to investigate 2 models of colorectal cancer significantly inhibited formation of intestinal tumors in both models. In Apc1638+/- mice and Muc2-/- mice, the tumor incidence was reduced by 45% and 50%, respectively, and tumor multiplicity was decreased by 60% and 50%, respectively. The mechanistic evidence indicates that tumors in the Apc1638+/- mice were inhibited by suppressing beta-catenin signaling, while the Muc2-/- mice tumor suppression was a resulted from decreasing chronic inflammation. While proliferation of intestinal cells from both models was inhibited, cell differentiation was not changed in either.[45]

Since ulcerative colitis can dramatically increase the risk of colon cancers, a model in mice of ulcerative colitis induced by dextran sodium sulfate was studied in conjunction with diets of 5% or 10% freeze-dried black raspberry powder for 7-14 days and compared to controls. The berry powder greatly reduced acute injury and ulceration to the colon epithelium by the dextran, as key pro-inflammatory cytokines including IL-1β and TNF-α were suppressed for up to 7 days by the black raspberries. Colonic COX-2 and plasma PGE_2 were markedly decreased the latter, from 276 in controls to 34 ng/ml.[4]

IN VITRO

Using a colon cancer cell proliferation model to investigate the differences between 7 Ohio growing site locations, 3 cultivar varieties (Bristol, Jewel, MacBlack), and 3 fruit maturity stages (underripe, ripe, overripe), 75 black raspberry freeze-dried extracts in concentrations of 0.6 and 1.2 mg/ml were evaluated in HT-29 cell cultures using 96-well plates. Cell proliferation was significantly reduced by all extracts in a dose-dependent manner, but the effect was influenced significantly by the 3 variables studied (location, variety, maturity), independent of total phenolic and total monomeric anthocyanin content. This illustrates the complexity of the interactive phytochemical influences of black raspberries, including ellagic acid, flavonols, and phenolic acids.[46]

Total monomeric anthocyanins differed significantly in juice samples from 1 growing site (higher than the 6 others), 2 cultivars (Jewel > MacBlack), and all 3 maturity stages (overripe > ripe > underripe). Total phenolics in the juices varied significantly in the same growing site (higher) and stages of maturity (overripe > ripe > underripe), but not between cultivars. For the solid phase extracts (SPE), only the stages of maturity showed significant differences in total phenolics (overripe > underripe) and total monomeric anthocyanins (overripe, ripe > underripe).[46]

Colon cancer cell inhibition was significantly greater with the SPE of berries from one growing site than from another site. (The site with the lowest inhibition from SPE also had the highest phenolics and anthocyanins in its juice.) The SPE from Bristol and Jewel cultivars caused significantly greater inhibition that the MacBlack SPE. The underripe berry SPE produced significantly greater inhibition than those from the ripe and the overripe berries. These results with the SPE were consistent with both concentrations tested.[46]

A metabolomic investigation of black raspberry phytochemical components' antiproliferative activity against the colon cancer cell line HT-29 used partial least-square regression analysis to develop a statistical model. This model identified individual component's relative contribution to inhibiting cancer cell proliferation. Using this model, cyanidin 3-xylosylrutinoside and cyanidin 3-rutinoside were identified as the major bioactivity contributors. However, derivatives of salicylic acid, citric acid, and methyl ellagic acid, along with quercetin 3-rutinoside, quercetin 3-glucoside, p-coumaric acid, and epicatechin were also significant contributors to the berry's antiproliferative activity.[47] This model clearly demonstrates the complexity of berry bioactivity in the context of the combination multiple components contributing to the beneficial effect.

REDUCING MAMMARY CARCINOGENESIS AND INCREASING BREAST CANCER CELL RADIOSENSITIVITY

IN ANIMALS

In a study of female rats given a 17β-estradiol implant, a control diet or diets with 400 ppm ellagic acid or 1% or 2.5% black raspberry were given 2 weeks before the estrogen and 6, 18, or 24 weeks afterward. The ellagic acid and 1% black raspberry and 2.5% black raspberry diets significantly reduced mammary tumor incidence 19%, 19%, and 13%, tumor volume 65%, 44%, and 67%, and tumor multiplicity 41%, 43.5%, and 51%, respectively, 24 weeks after the estrogen implant.[48]

In these groups, after 6 weeks the implanted controls had a 48-fold increase in CYP1A1, but this was significantly attenuated to 12-fold by the 2.5% black raspberry diet. This berry diet also significantly reduced CYP1B1 expression by 6-fold after 6 weeks, and the 5-fold induction of 17β-hydroxysteroid dehydrogenase was significantly reduced to about 2-fold by both the black raspberry and ellagic acid supplemented diets. After 18 weeks, these supplemental diets reversed the 2-fold induction of catechol-O-methyl transferase expression, and after 24 weeks, the 2.5% black raspberry diet significantly reduced CYP1A1 induction. Since steroid receptor effects of estradiol were not altered by the supplemental diets, this suggests the reductions in mammary tumors were associated with suppressing estrogen-metabolizing enzymes early in estrogen-induced carcinogenesis.[48]

In a follow-up study of rats given the 17β-estradiol implant to induce tumors of the mammary glands, besides a control diet the animals were given diets with 5% freeze-dried black raspberries. Ellagic acid was detected at 97-294 ng/ml in the plasma of rats fed the black raspberries. Mammary tumor appearance occurred in controls at 84 days, but this was significantly delayed by 39 days with the black raspberry diet. In addition to tumor latency being delayed by the black raspberry diet, it also downregulated estrogen receptor-α expression.[49]

IN VITRO

Before or after exposure of MCF-7 breast adenocarcinoma cells to ionizing radiation, the cells in culture were exposed to black raspberry methanol extract containing anthocyanins but not ellagic acid. The cells were harvested 1, 3, 6, 24, 48, and 72 hours after the radiation exposure and tested for expression of transcriptional regulators. The extract inhibited NF-κB activation in a dose-dependent manner, as well as its sustained activation. In addition, TNF-α, IL-1α, and manganese superoxide dismutase levels were all inhibited. Breast cancer cell survival was suppressed by the berry extract, and MCF-7 cell death was enhanced. These results indicate that the black raspberry anthocyanins may be potent as a radiosensitizer in breast cancer cells.[50]

PROTECTION FROM SOLAR AND IONIZING RADIATION

IN ANIMALS

When hairless mice were exposed to a minimal erythemal dose of ultraviolet-B (UVB) radiation 3 times weekly on nonconsecutive days for 25 weeks, they were treated topically after each exposure with either an 80% ethanolic black raspberry extract or the vehicle. The berry extract significantly reduced the skin tumor number and average size compared to controls, beginning at week 19. In an acute UVB exposure, the extract, when applied topically, significantly reduced the edema, oxidative DNA damage, p53 protein levels, and neutrophil activation after 48 hours.[51]

IN VITRO

When mouse epidermal cells were exposed to a methanol extract fraction from black raspberries, it inhibited UVB-induced activation of of pro-inflammatory NF-κB, but not AP-1, in a time- and dose-dependent manner. Cyanin-3-rutinoside contributed to the effect. Methanolic fractions from strawberries or blueberries did not contain this compound, and neither inhibited the NF-κB activation.[52]

OTHER ANTICANCER MECHANISMS OF FRACTIONS AND COMPONENTS

IN VITRO

Inhibiting angiogenesis is a major means of reducing tumor growth and limiting metastasis as a complementary approach to controlling cancer. Reducing the new growth of blood vessels stifles expansion of cancer by reducing nutrients and oxygen to the malignant tissue. An extract of black raspberry was shown to be anti-angiogenic in a model using human tissue. The anti-angiogenic fraction was completely effective at 0.075% in preventing new vessel initiation and growth, but this fraction is only 1% of the weight of fresh whole black raspberries. One of the active compounds in this fraction is gallic acid, but the subfractions were not more potent than the whole fraction.[53]

The cyanidin-3-rutinoside extracted and purified from black raspberry was tested in human leukemia and lymphoma cell lines. It was shown to activate caspase-3 and -9 and induce apoptosis in leukemic HL-60 myeloblastic cells in a time- and dose-dependent manner, based on the intracellular accumulation of peroxides. Likewise, it induced apoptosis in human lymphoblastic MOLT-4, Daudi, and CCRF-CEM cell lines in a dose-dependent manner. It also activated reactive oxygen species (ROS)-dependent c-Jun N-terminal kinase (JNK) and p38 mitogen-activated protein kinase (MAPK) that contributed to mitochondrial release of apoptogenic factors and cell death. This anthocyanin did not increase accumulation of ROS in normal human peripheral blood mononuclear cells but reduced intracellular peroxide levels in these, nor did it produce cytotoxic effects on such cells. Thus, in the tested human white blood cell cultures cyanidin-3-rutinoside was found to be selectively active against leukemia cells.[54]

METABOLIC SYNDROME

In a randomized, placebo-controlled study to investigate the influence of black raspberry, known for its antioxidant and anti-inflammatory activities, on patients with metabolic syndrome, a freeze-dried water extract of the unripe fruit was used in doses of 750 mg daily for 12 weeks. A group of 39 patients with metabolic syndrome took the black raspberry as 4 capsules daily, while 38 were assigned to placebo. After 12 weeks the black raspberry group, compared to placebo, had significantly lowered total cholesterol and cholesterol/HDL ratio. Also, the cytokines IL-6, TNF-α, and adiponectin were reduced significant reduced in the extract group compared to placebo. Likewise, flow-mediated dilation of the brachial artery was significantly increased. These finding suggest benefits for the cholesterol, inflammatory, and blood flow components of metabolic syndrome.[55]

COMPARATIVE VALUE AND QUALITY OF FREEZE-DRIED POWDER, EXTRACTS, AND DERIVATIVES

Human and animals studies have mostly used freeze-dried black raspberry powder in studying cancer prevention. Whether using the powder, extracts, fractions, or isolated anthocyanins or ellagic acid, there has been little or no toxicity problems with oral administration. The advantages of using the whole freeze-dried berry are several. They contain multiple chemopreventive agents, while the extracts lose some berry content variety and quantity, and anthocyanin fractions or isolates lack ellagic acid contributions and vice versa. The whole berry powder is relatively inexpensive in comparison to extracts and especially the anthocyanin isolates. Stability is generally diminished as components become more concentrated in extracts or as isolates.[6]

In an attempt to design easily consumed forms of black raspberry powder for a long-term prevention trial on prostate cancer, 3 types of preparations were formulated. A confection with 20% freeze-dried black raspberry powder, 29.5% sugar, 11% corn syrup, 38% water, 1% pectin, and 0.5% citric acid and 2 nectars (viscous juice) with 4% or 8% powder, 3% sugar, 1% corn syrup, 91% or 87% water, and 1% pectin. After large-scale processing the confection retained 94% of anthocyanins, 96% ellagitannins, and 106% of ellagic acid (some from ellagitannins), while the 4% and 8% nectars retained 86% or 69% anthocyannins, 66% or 91% ellagitannins, and 114% or 128% of total ellagic acid, respectively. The ellagitannins and ellagic acid were almost completely retained in both forms after 8 weeks of storage, whereas anthocyanins diminished in the confection by 11% and in the 4%

and 8% nectars by 10% and 4%, respectively. Both forms were well-accepted for their palatibility.[56]

A disadvantage of whole berry powder is the difficulty to standardize content, and consumption of much larger doses are generally needed. Contamination of berries with chemicals or microbes are possible, comparable to concerns with other commercial fruits and vegetables. Extracts are more difficult to prepare, but smaller doses are necessary. Isolated anthocyanins are difficult to synthesize, have poor bioavailability, and therefore can still require substantial oral doses. The target tissue helps determine the preferred form, as whole powder provides good exposure to alimenary tissue, while extracts are more practical for external applications to the skin.[6]

Since most of its commercial growth is limited to Oregon, extensive demand for black raspberry's health benefits has challenged the limited supply. This has led to its adulteration in many dietary supplement products. Because black raspberry has a distinct anthocyanin profile from blackberry, red raspberry, or any other *Rubus* species berry, it is relatively simple to differentiate it by phytochemical assays. In a 2014 study of 19 commercially-available black raspberry products, either freeze-dried whole berries, powdered berries, or berry extracts, the composition and concentration of their anthocyanins was analyzed. The cost of preparations in capsules ranged from 6 cents to 79 cents per capsule; both of the products at these price range extremes were apparently spurious, containing no black raspberry anthocyanins.[57]

> Because black raspberry has a distinct anthocyanin profile from blackberry, red raspberry, or any other *Rubus* species berry, it is relatively simple to differentiate it by phytochemical assays.[57]

Three of the 19 contained no anthocyanins at all, while another 4 had no anthocyanins characteristic of black raspberry. Aside from these 7, the other 12 had a wide range of black raspberry anthocyanin content with cyanidin-3-rutinoside as the main anthocyanin. Six of these (3 loose powder, 2 in capsules, 1 liquid extract) had all 7 of the anthocyanins found in black raspberry. These 6 products also had the greatest total anthocyanin contents ranging from 828.5 to 1742.2 mg/100 g for powders and capsules and 2904 mg/100 g for the only liquid extract analyzed. The other 6 products had 5 of the 7 anthocyanins with very low total anthocyanin contents from 18.1 to 114.8 mg/100 g.[57]

MECHANISMS OF ELLAGIC ACID REDUCTION OF CARCINOGENESIS

IN ANIMALS

The main importance of ellagic acid is its contribution to the inhibition of carcinogenesis. This has been shown in mice by feeding of ellagic acid in drinking water for 16 weeks which reduces phase I metabolic bioactivation of the procarcinogen benzo[a]pyene. Its effects include decreasing liver and lung cytochrome P450 (CYP) levels by 20-25% and increasing phase II elimination of reactive intermediates by enhanced glutathione S-transferase (GST) activity.[58]

Likewise, after 23 days rats fed ellagic acid showed a 25% decrease in liver and esophageal CYP levels, while phase II enzyme levels of GST, NAD(P)H:quinone reductase (QR), and UDP-glucuronosyl transferase (UGT) in the liver were increased 26%, 17%, and 75%, respectively.[59] Rats fed ellagic acid also had significant increases in liver GST activity and GST-Ya mRNA content. This specific increase in detoxification potential can reduce carcinogen-induced mutagenesis and tumorigensis.[60] Similarly, feeding rats ellagic acid increased the activity of liver QR by 9-fold and of lung QR by 2-fold, while liver QR mRNA was increased 8-fold.[61]

As a means of preventing cancer, the reduction of DNA damage is paramount. Ellagic acid is one berry component that has been shown to reduce oxidative DNA adducts. Feeding ellagic acid at 400 ppm or supplementing the diet with 5% whole dried berries that are low (blueberry), medium (strawberry), or high (red raspberry) in ellagic acid to mice, the blueberry and strawberry diets resulted in a moderate 25% reduction of DNA adducts. On the other hand, the raspberry and ellagic acid diets resulted in significant reductions of 59% and 48%, respectively, and a 3- to 8-fold over-expression of genes involved in DNA repair. These findings suggest that ellagic acid plays a significant role in reducing oxidative DNA damage and may increase DNA repair.[62]

> Findings suggest that ellagic acid plays a significant role in reducing oxidative DNA damage and may increase DNA repair.[62]

In Vitro

Examining the effects of benzo[a]pyrene with or without ellagic acid or different fractions from freeze-dried strawberries (*Fragara ananassa*) and Pacific black raspberries (*R. ursinus*) in the Syrian hamster embryo cell transformation model after 1 or 7 days, the ellagic acid and the polar methanolic fractions of both berries not containing ellagic acid produced dose-dependent decreases in transformation compared to benzopyrene alone. This appears to be due to berry polar fractions inhibiting the initiation stage and ellagic acid interference with both the initiation and promotion stages of carcinogenesis. These effects may involve uptake, activation, and/or detoxification of the procarcinogen benzopyrene and/or impacting its DNA binding or the DNA repair.[63] Anticarcinogenic, antimutagenic, and/or antitumorigenic effects of ellagic acid have been documented with a variety of other carcinogens as well (aflatoxin B_1, nitroso compunds, 3-methylcholanthrene, N-2-fluorenylacetamide) in tissue cultures from mice, rats, and humans.[64]

Mechanisms for Ellagic Acid Reducing Liver Toxicity from Alcohol

In Animals

The component ellagic acid at 60 mg/kg has been shown to reduce effects of alcohol liver toxicity in rats induced by ethanol given orally for 45 days at 7.9 g/kg daily.[65,66,67] This involves decreasing expressions of liver fibrotic markers, including matrix metalloproteinases and tissue inhibitors of metalloproteinase, by acting as an antifibrotic agent.[65] The same dosage improved body weight and circulatory nonenzymatic antioxidant status of vitamins C and E and reduced glutathione. Enzymatic antioxidants superoxide dismutase, glutathione peroxidase, and catalase were likewise positively modulated.[66] This ellagic acid dose in rats also reduced liver marker enzymes AST, ALT, GGT, and alkaline phosphatase, while it decreased cholesterol, triglyceride, and free fatty acid levels that were significantly elevated by alcohol.[66,67] It also decreased plasma indices of lipid peroxidation.[67] These studies suggest that ellagic acid may be of benefit in treating liver conditions caused by alcohol abuse.[65,66,67]

These studies suggest that ellagic acid may be of benefit in treating liver conditions caused by alcohol abuse.[65,66,67]

SUMMARY

The consistent effect of freeze-dried black raspberries *in vivo* has been to reduce the development of cancer from precancerous conditions or induced by carcinogenic substances. Some *in vivo* evidence also suggests the potential to inhibit the growth of established colon cancer cells. A number of phenolic components apparently contribute to these effects including anthocyanins characteristic of black raspberry such as cyanidin-3-rutinoside, as well as phenolic acids, especially ellagic acid. The bioavailability of the anthocyanins is limited by their absorption, causing them to be particularly effective for their local effects in reducing cancer development along the alimentary tract from the mouth to the rectum. The ellagic acid, on the other hand, appears to provide better systemic protection.

Like other berries high in anthocyanins and antioxidant capacity, black raspberry appears to help protect against the conditions associated with metabolic syndrome. Yet, regarding its chemopreventive activity, no single component or extract fraction has been able to duplicate the efficacy of the whole berry, since multiple components with different mechanisms contribute to the overall effect. The challenge of obtaining an authentic black raspberry product is complicated by the number of products in the commercial market that are spurious (about one third) and diluted/adulterated (another third). While cost can be one indication of quality, since authentic black raspberry products are relatively expensive, high cost is no assurance of quality or authenticity. Much of the chemopreventive research on freeze-dried black raspberries has been done with topical oral application by humans or oral consumption by humans and animals, showing that eating the berries is a flavorful and effective way of enjoying the health benefits of this powerful food.

Black Chokeberry

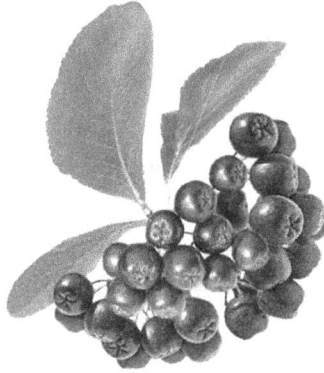

CHOKEBERRY AND ITS EXTRACTS AND/OR JUICE CONTAIN ANTIOXIDANT POLYPHENOLICS SHOWN TO BENEFICIALLY IMPACT CARDIOVASCULAR FUNCTION. BESIDES SUPPORTING VITAL ORGAN FUNCTIONS, CHOKEBERRIES HELP WARD OFF INFECTIONS AND HAVE ANTI-INFLAMMATORY, ANTIMUTAGENIC, AND ANTICANCER PROPERTIES TO BETTER MAINTAIN NORMAL CELL AND TISSUE GROWTH. PRELIMINARY EVIDENCE FROM CLINICAL TRIALS WITH TEST PREPARATIONS HIGH IN ANTHOCYANINS SUGGESTS ITS BENEFITS ARE PRIMARILY FROM ALLEV-IATION OF OXIDATIVE STRESS, ESPECIALLY AMONG THOSE SUFFERING FROM METABOLIC SYNDROME.

Black chokeberry (*Aronia melanocarpa*) is native from the Great Lakes region to the northeastern USA, into southeastern Canada and south in the higher Appalchian Mountain elevations. It grows best in full sun and moist soil with annual precipitation of 15 inches or more. The black chokeberry shrub usually grow from 3 to 12 feet. Its leaves, noteworthy in autumn for their vivid red color, are simple and alternate with pinnate venation and raised glands on the top midrib. The 5-petaled white flowers are small and grouped in corymbs of 10-25. These produce small clusters of berries.

Its pome fruit are pea-size with 1-5 small seeds but quite juicy.

The berries shrivel up and begin dropping shortly after ripening. Black chokeberries are quite astringent, largely due to procyanidins, and are used to color and flavor beverages and food products. The astringency also helps protect it from pests including insects and microbes, but the berries are consumed by wild birds including grouse. Several commercial cultivars have been developed in America.

Referred to henceforth simply as chokeberry, the fruit was used traditionally by the Forest Potawatomi tribe of Native Americans to treat colds. It has been shown to provide immune enhancement plus antiviral and antibacterial activities. Nonetheless, native use has long been overshadowed by development of commercial cultivation, especially in Russia and eastern Europe for making jam, juice, and wine. Its widespread cultivation began in the former Soviet Union in the 1940s. Chokeberry's value for promoting health is largely due to its antioxidative activity, including stomach- and liver-protecting properties, besides having antidiabetic, lipid-lowering, and platelet-inhibiting effects.[1] Repeated clinical findings include increases in antioxidant enzymes, normalization of oxidized LDL levels, and reductions in total cholesterol, blood sugar, and blood pressure.[2,3]

CHOKEBERRY POLYPHENOLICS VERSUS ITS POMACE AND JUICE

Chokeberry's main polyphenolic components (up to 8% dry weight [dw]) include anthocyanins ($\leq$ 2% dw) and procyanidins ($\leq$ 5% dw).[1] Chokeberry's unusually high polyphenol content was well assessed in a study comparing freeze-dried fruit, pomace (the material left after juice is expressed from the fruit), and juice. The research findings show large amounts of polyphenols are left behind after juicing. In some cases, due to reductions in weight of other content (e.g, sugar and fiber extracted with the juice) or from enhanced polymerization (e.g., procyanidins), the relative content in the pomace of certain specific polyphenols and total polyphenols increased by percentage of weight compared to the fruit, which led to greater antioxidant activity for the pomace than for the juice or even the original fruit.[4]

The research findings show large amounts of polyphenols are left behind after juicing.[4]

The relative percentages of polyphenols therefore vary between these 3 forms of chokeberry preparations, i.e., berries, pomace, and juice, measured as milligrams per 100 grams freeze-dried weight. For instance, the yields of procyanidins for these 3 preparations were 5.2%, 8.2%, and 1.6% dw, respectively, while anthocyanin contents were 2.0%, 1.8%, and 1.2% dw, respectively. Of the less abundant polyphenols, the relative yields of these 3 forms for chlorogenic plus neochlorogenic acid were 0.59%, 0.37%, and 0.80% dw and for quercetin glycosides plus derivatives were 0.10%, 0.17%, and 0.16% dw, respectively.[4]

POLYPHENOLIC AND ANTIOXIDANT COMPARISONS BETWEEN BERRIES

Chokeberry has been gaining increasing attention in research in conditions associated with oxidative stress. Based on its greater antioxidant capacity as measured by ORAC in comparison with other more common commercial berries and fruits, it exceeds elderberry, blueberries, blackberry, black currant, lingonberry, red currant, red raspberry, strawberry, cranberry, orange, grapes, and apples (in decreasing order) and juices such as pomegranate, blueberry, black cherry, cranberry, orange and apple (in decreasing order, as measured by TEAC) and red wine.[5]

In a test comparing phytochemical contents of 8 wild and 17 cultivated berries including various species of *Fragaria, Ribes, Rubus,* and *Vaccinium* along with *Lycium, Morus, Rosa, Sorbus,* and *Sambucus* species, chokeberry had by far the highest quantity of total phenols (10,132 mg gallic acid equivalents/kg). The next highest in total phenolic content were rowanberry (*Sorbus aucuparia*; 5407 GAE/kg), wild elderberry (*Sambucus nigra*; 5149 GAE/kg), dog rose (*Rosa canina*; 4773 GAE/kg), American cranberry (4522 GAE/kg) and wild strawberry (*Fragaria vesca*; 4347 GAE/kg). Strawberries, raspberries, and blackberries grown in the wild had 2-5 times more total phenolics than when cultivated.[6]

Including various species of *Fragaria, Ribes, Rubus,* and *Vaccinium* along with *Lycium, Morus, Rosa, Sorbus,* and *Sambucus* species, chokeberry had by far the highest quantity of total phenols.[6]

A few other comparative studies help to further illustrate this point on the relatively higher antioxidant potency of chokeberry compared to other berries. In testing the anthocyanin and proanthocyanidin contents of black currant (*Ribes nigrum*), red currant (*Ribes rubrum*), gooseberries (*Ribes grossularia*), elderberry (*Sambucus nigra*), and chokeberry, the chokeberry had the highest concentration of total anthocyanins (1.5 g/100 g fresh weight [fw], in proportions of 10 parts cyanidin 3-galactoside to 4 parts cyanidin 3-arabinoside to 0.5 parts cyanidin 3-xyloside to 0.4 parts cyanidin 3-glucoside) and the highest total proanthocyanidin content (664 mg/100 g fw, predominantly procyanidins). The total antioxidant capacity as measured by lipophilic and hydrophilic ORAC was likewise greatest in chokeberry (161 mcmol TE/g fw), paralleling the phenolic content.[7] Chokeberry is also noted for its high phenolic acid content, second only to rowanberry among 12 common commercial berries and fruits tested.[5]

Comparisons made in polyphenolic content and antioxidant activities between 70% ethanolic extracts of chokeberry and highbush blueberry revealed that the chokeberry extract had 4 times the total phenolics, 3 times the total flavonoids, and 9 times the proanthocyanidin content as these blueberries. This translated to significantly greater free radical-scavenging activity at 500 mcg/ml extract *in vitro*; with 2,2-diphenyl-1-picrylhydrazyl (DPPH) the activity of chokeberry extract was 72.7% versus 40.6% for blueberry extract, and for 2,2'-azino-bis(3-ethylbenzothiazoline-6-sulphonic acid (ABTS) the activities were 46.3% versus 8.6%, respectively. The antioxidant reducing power for chokeberry extract in the ferric reducing ability of plasma (FRAP) assay at 500 mcg/ml was also significantly greater than for blueberry extract. Thus, the activities of the extracts correlates with the phenolic contents.[8]

While the bilberry and rabbiteye blueberry *Vaccinium* species each each contain 15 different anthocyanins, black currant has 6, and elderberry and chokeberry have 4 major anthocyanins each. Though held in common with bilberry and rabbiteye and highbush blueberries, chokeberry's yield of cyanidin 3-galactoside and cyanidin 3-arabinoside are both much greater than in these *Vaccinium* species.[8,9] All of these berries are potent DPPH radical scavengers; elderberry is the least potent, though it has the highest total anthocyanin content of which most is the unique cyanidin 3-sambubioside.[9] Chokeberry and blueberry juices were also the second and fourth most potent beverages, respectively, of the 35 tested, including 10 other fruit juices, for inhibiting the sulfotransferase activity in Caco-2 cells *in vitro*.[10]

While anthocyanins are major antioxidant components in chokeberry and *Vaccinium* species berries, the phenolic proportions differ by species and cultivars. In wild chokeberry cyanidin 3-galactoside and cyanidin 3-arabinoside along with caffeic acid and its derivatives are in very high concentrations and contribute the most antioxidant activity. Highbush blueberry cultivar Sierra's predominant antioxidant phenolic is the caffeic acid derivative chlorogenic acid and to a lesser extent delphinidin 3-galactoside and other anthocyanidins. Lingonberry (*V. vitis-idaea*) cultivar Amberland contains cyanidin 3-galactoside as its most important antioxidant with important additions by quercetin glycosides. For cranberry cultivar Ben Lear peonidin 3-galactoside and its other glycosides stand out. The total ORAC values for these 4 berry representatives, respectively, were 95.1, 22.8, 12.8, and 9.2 mcmole/g.[11]

Another study compared the total polyphenols, anthocyanins, and reduced ascorbic acid in black currants, red currants, European blackberries (*Rubus fruticosus*), red raspberries (*Rubus idaeus*), and chokeberries. Again, chokeberries were found to have the highest content of total polyphenols (690 mg/100 g fresh weight) and total anthocyanins (460 mg/100 g fresh weight), with black currants in a relatively close second place. Black currants had by far the highest ascorbic acid content, while chokeberry was similar to the other berries. When the radical scavenging activity for quenching 50% of the DPPH radical in solution was tested, chokeberry showed the most potency by having the lowest effective concentration with black currant again in second.[12]

Comparing the total phenolics and antioxidant activity of 70% aqueous acetone extracts of 13 berries and 80% aqueous methanolic extracts of 8 vegetables and 32 medicinal herbs, the berry extracts had the greatest phenolic contents and antioxidant effects. For phenolics, chokeberry was only second to crowberry (*Empetrum nigrum*) among the berries and a close third among all extracts of berries, vegetables, and herbs following purple loosestrife (*Lythrum salicaria*). In antioxidant activity crowberry, chokeberry, rowanberry, and all *Rubus* and *Vaccinium* species (except for red raspberry and bilberry, respectively) provided greater than 87% inhibition of MeLo oxidation at 500 ppm and 5000 ppm (chokeberry was 93-94%).[13]

CHOKEBERRY CULTIVATION AND PHENOLIC CONTENT

Comparing different *Aronia* species for polyphenolic content shows that on a dry weight basis black chokeberry (*A. melanocarpa*) has the highest anthocyanin yield (3.4-14.8 mg/g), mostly cyanidin-3-galactoside, whereas red chokeberry (*A. arbutifolia*) has the lowest. The red berry species has the highest proanthocyanin content, while purple chokeberry (*A. prunifolia*) has the highest yield of chlorogenic acids. Non-anthocyanin flavonoid content was comparable between species.[14] Regarding the relative contributions of these polyphenols to the antiradical activity of black chokeberry, as determined by reducing initial DPPH concentration by 50%, anthocyanins had the greatest effect with a 56.3% contribution, followed by proanthocyanidins and insoluble phenols at 34.8%, with flavonols and phenolic acids contributing just 8.9%.[15]

Though the anthocyanins and oligomeric proanthocyanidins were similar in wild berries from Illinois and in cultivated berries from Europe, the wild berries had a higher total flavonoid content, while the cultivated berries had up to 67% more nonphenolic compounds.[16] Agricultural means of increasing the phenolic components have been investigated. Fruit of 10-year-old chokeberry plants of the Nero variety grown in the Czech Republic were analyzed for pigment content, and the results in g/kg dry weight were 37.7 phenolics, 6.4 anthocyanins, 0.66 flavonoids, and 0.35 quercetin. Ethanolamine phosphate, an ornithine decarboxylase (ODC) inhibitor that reduces polyamine biosynthesis, when applied to the foliage in mid-July increased phenolics by 15% and anthocyanins by 23.6%, while also significantly increasing flavonoids and quercetin. This indicates that this ODC inhibitor greatly increases phenolic pigment synthesis.[17]

Though the anthocyanins and oligomeric proanthocyanidins were similar in wild berries from Illinois and in cultivated berries from Europe, the wild berries had a higher total flavonoid content.[16]

The chokeberry cultivar 'Viking' grown in Sweden was studied to see how fertilizer application affected berry yield, weight, anthocyanins, and other content. Though fertilizers increased vegetative growth and berry yield, it decreased by weight the anthocyanin content and total acidity of the berries. Berry weight and specific anthocyanin composition remained unchanged.[18]

IMPACT OF PROCESSING AND/OR STORAGE ON JUICE AND SOLID EXTRACTS

Chokeberry fruit juice that had been filtered, pasteurized at 80°C for 10 minutes and stored at 0°C was found to still have potent antiradical activity *in vitro*, likely due to antioxidant effects of the phenolic constituents.[19] The polyphenols in fresh frozen chokeberries were studied in the context of juicing, processing, and storage. After the berry mash was heated to 95°C, depectinized, and pressed, the nonclaried juice was pasteurized at 90°C, bottled, and stored for 1-6 months at room temperature. Anthocyanins were lost during juicing, due to removal of skins and seeds after pressing. Thermal treatments further degraded the anthocyanins, during which protocatechuic acid increased. Further anthocyanin losses occured linearly during storage due to conversion to polymeric forms. On the other hand, flavonols, hydroxycinnamic acids, and total proanthocyanidins were all retained in the juice and during the 6-month storage.[20]

In assessing the best method(s) for preserving phenolic compounds and antioxidant capacity when drying the juice to form powder, spray drying was found to be most effective. Though the differences in total polyphenols were not significant, spray drying gave significantly higher amounts of flavonoids, total monomeric anthocyanins, cyanidin-

3-glucoside, and total proanthocyanins than the other 2 methods. Freeze-drying was the next best method for drying the juice and was significantly better than oven vacuum drying at 40º-80ºC for total proanthocyanidins. Freeze-drying was likewise significantly better than 80ºC vacuum drying for preserving monomeric anthocyanins and cyanidin-3-glucoside and than 40ºC and 80ºC oven drying for FRAP antioxidant power.[21]

In a comparative study of chokeberry preparations, 4 liquid juice products (recommended dose 100 ml), 1 syrup (recommended dose 20 ml), and 1 solid extract (450 mg capsule; 8-10:1 berry pomace to extract; 50% ethanolic solvent) were analyzed for anthocyanin content. The extract and syrup yielded much lower total anthocyanins than 3 of the 4 juices. To obtain the estimated 110 mg of anthocyanins daily that provides an effective amount for treating metabolic syndrome, the required daily doses of solid extract and syrup would be 18 g and 740 ml, respectively. For the juices, the daily doses to achieve the desired anthocyanin intake were 100, 150, 330, and 1860 ml. Thus, for addressing metabolic syndrome reasonable daily doses were provided by 3 of the 6 products. However, for treating influenza with 3.5 g of anthocyanins daily, none of these chokeberry products were deemed adequate for providing an appropriate dose.[22]

Analysis of a Polish pharmaceutical chokeberry fruit solid extract dietary supplement revealed a total polyphenolic content of 61-64% with 16-17% total anthocyanins. The slight variations were due to differences in dilution, filtration, and light exposure storage conditions.[23] A 450 mg capsule of this extract would yield 74 mg of total anthocyanins; thus, apparently 1.5 capsules could provide the daily dose of 110 mg anthocyanins for treating metabolic syndrome.

ANTHOCYANIN METABOLISM AND BIOAVAILABILITY AND POLYPHENOL BIOCONVERSION

IN HUMANS

Absorption of the anthocyanins in chokeberry juice was tested in 13 human volunteers. The dose was individualized to provide 0.8 mg anthocyanins per kg body weight, and cyanidin-3-galactoside made up

66% of the total anthocyanins. The maximum plasma concentration of 32.7 nmol/L from 8 cyanidin derivatives occurred 1.3 hours after consumption. Urinary excretion was greatest during the first 2 hours, but only 0.25% of the cyanidin metabolites were excreted in the urine in the first 24 hours.[24]

IN ANIMALS

When an anthocyanin-rich extract of chokeberry was fed to rats for 14 weeks at 26 mg/kg body weight, anthocyanin peaks were significant in the urine and in fecal extracts, compared to controls. Even though anthocyanins were detected in the serum, quantities were not measurable.[25]

In comparing the absorption of different anthocyanins based on the cyanidin sugar moiety, freeze-dried powders of chokeberry, elderberry, and black currant were fed once to weanling pigs. The relative proportion of anthocyanins in chokeberry is 66% cyanidin-3-galactoside, 28% cyanidin-3-arabinoside, 4% cyanidin-3-xyloside, and 2% cyanidin-3-glucoside. All 4 cyanidin anthocyanins from chokeberry were subject to methylation and glucuronidation, undergoing phase I and II metabolism in pigs. Anthocyanins with delphinidin were not metabolized, and those with rutinose or sambublose from black currant or elderberry were mostly excreted intact, as were the anthocyanins with 2 or 3 attached sugars. So, both the sugar and the aglycone components of the molecules influence absorption and metabolism of anthocyanins.[26]

The relative proportion of anthocyanins in chokeberry is 66% cyanidin-3-galactoside, 28% cyanidin-3-arabinoside, 4% cyanidin-3-xyloside, and 2% cyanidin-3-glucoside.[26]

Anthocyanin absorption appears to be poor, but it varies between species due to differences in metabolism and/or bacterial degradation. Conjugation likely affects the biological activity of anthocyanins. Still, anthocyanins appear to play an important role in the reported health benefits of chokeberry. Proanthocyanidins are unlikely to be absorbed intact due to their high molecular weight and polymeric nature, but though no *in vivo* bioavailability study has thus-far been conducted on these chokeberry-isolated components, they are believed to be converted, in part, to well-absorbed phenolic acids. Neochlorogenic and chlorogenic acids in chokeberry are naturally esterified, impairing their conversion and absorption in humans. The potent antioxidant quercetin glycosides and epicatechin have been shown in studies from other sources to be absorbed (after the glycoside hydrolyzation), but their content in chokeberry is relatively low.[2]

IN VITRO

Chokeberry juice was exposed to simulated digestion in the presence of food paste consisting of 10% carbohydrates, 3% protein, and 1% fat to assess the effects on polyphenols and the antioxidant activity. The 4.5 ml of juice was combined with 6 ml artificial saliva and 4.5 g of food matrix, then exposed to 12 ml gastric juice at pH 2, incubated 1 hour and then mixed with 12 ml intestinal juice and 6 ml of bile at pH 5.4. Compared with juice diluted proportionally with water, digested juice had lower polyphenolics (373 mcg vs. 253 mcg, respectively), while a 10-fold decrease in proanthocyanins was observed (from 34.2 to 3.33 mg/100 ml, respectively). Radical scavenging activity and total reducing power were each reduced about 45%. Still, when exposed to Caco-2 human colon adenocarcinoma cell culture, the digested juice reduced the proliferation rate by about 25% compared to controls.[27] It seems probable that local effects of unabsorbed proanthocyanidins in the colon would be beneficial.[2]

Chokeberry wine high in polyphenols was tested alone under conditions that simulate digestive exposure in the stomach with pepsin for 4 hr. at pH 2.0, then exposure to pancreatic juice and bile in small intestine conditions plus intestinal microflora at 37°C for 2.5 hr. at pH 7.4, followed by anaerobic conditions of the colon at 37°C for 18 hr. at pH 8.0. While p-coumaric acid content was relatively unaffected by these changes, chlorogenic acid decreased dramatically from the stomach to small intestine conditions. Caffeic acid content was reduced with the change from small intestine to the colon. Paradoxically, trans-resveratrol doubled from the stomach to the small intestine conditions, then returned to stomach levels under the colon conditions. While the antioxidant capacity was gradually and significantly reduced from stomach through colon conditions, the total polyphenol content dropped significantly after small intestine exposure and precipitously after colon simulation. The intestinal microflora showed a considerable diminishment after small intestine conditions for *Bifidobacterium* and *Lactobacillus* and a precipitous one for *Enterobacteriaceae*, while *Enterococcus* showed considerable decreases after both small intestine and colon conditions.[28]

PROTECTION OF TISSUES FROM OXIDATIVE STRESS

IN HUMANS

When 150 ml of chokeberry juice with 35 mg anthocyanins was consumed daily for 1 month by rowers involved in ergometric exercise, blood samples taken 1 minute and 24 hours after the exercise test both showed significantly lower TBARS with the juice, while glutathione peroxidase was lower in the 1-minute sample and superoxide dismutase in the 24-hour sample of those taking the juice, compared to a placebo control group.[29]

In a randomized, placebo-controlled, double-blind study with 19 men on a national rowing team, 10 consumed 150 ml of chokeberry juice daily for 8 weeks. An ergometric test equivalent to rowing 2000 meters at the beginning and end of the study period showed that those consuming the juice had higher total antioxidant capacity and iron levels than controls. Those taking the juice also had significantly lower levels of the inflammatory cytokine TNF-α.[30]

In 11 healthy women with a "cold constitution", 150 mg/day of chokeberry dried hydro-ethanolic extract (35% anthocyanins) was taken as tablets after breakfast daily for 4 weeks. At the end of the trial, the body surface temperature was significantly higher than it was at baseline. Peripheral blood flow was not affected, even though plasma noradrenaline was significantly increased. Higher levels of urinary 8-hydroxy-2'-deoxyguanosine in 5 subjects at the beginning, an indication of oxidative stress, were significantly reduced at the end of the trial. Psychological factors related to cold feeling on the hand, foot, and hip were significantly improved. The effect appears to be due to increased noradrenaline and reduced oxidative stress.[31]

IN ANIMALS

A series of studies with rats has demonstrated that the antioxidative activity of chokeberry and its juice or its anthocyanin extracts protect against oxidative damage of different types in a variety of tissues. The damage to stomach mucosa from the anti-inflammatory drug indomethacin administered subcutaneously was significantly reduced when chokeberry juice was given orally 1 hour beforehand. The depth, number, area, and severity of the lesions were decreased, while gastric mucus production increased. The oxidative stress marker malondialdehyde (MDA) was reduced in the stomach and plasma dose-dependently by the juice.[32] A methanolic extract of the fruit given at a 2 g/kg body weight (b.w.) dose also reduced stomach mucosal damage from ethanol to less than 30% of the tissue damage in control rats, about the same protection as obtained with 100 mg/kg quercetin. A red pigment fraction including the anthocyanidin cyanidin 3-glucoside had a similar dose-dependent effect and at 30 mg/kg b.w. suppressed gastric mucosal damage by about 50%. Gastric acid secretion was not diminished.[33]

The damage to stomach mucosa from the anti-inflammatory drug indomethacin administered subcutaneously was significantly reduced when chokeberry juice was given orally 1 hour beforehand.[32]

Other evidence of reduced oxidative stress from juice intake involved rats given 10 ml/kg b.w. daily for 28 days. This reduced liver lipid peroxidation by 50% as expressed by thiobarbituric acid reactive substances (TBARS). In rats also given 150 mg/kg b.w. N-nitrosodiethylamine (NDEA) intraperitoneally, TBARS were reduced 53% by the juice, and DNA damage in leukocytes was reduced by 24%. The juice increased antioxidant enzyme activities for catalase, glutathione reductase, and gluthione peroxidase by 117%, 44%, and 56%, respectively, in rats given NDEA. In rats given 2 ml/kg b.w. carbon tetrachloride, TBARS were reduced 92% by the juice, and plasma protein carbonyls were decreased 55%.[34]

The liver in rats was again shown to be protected from damage due to carbon tetrachloride by short-term use of chokeberry juice. When the juice was given at 5-20 ml/kg b.w. for 2 days before and for 2 days with the liver toxin, necrotic changes were decreased dose-dependently along with significant reductions of liver and/or plasma levels of the lipid peroxidation marker MDA and the transaminase enzymes AST and ALT. The depletion of protective glutathione was also significantly reduced.[35] Cadmium is known to accumulate in the liver and kidneys and produce liver damage. When chokeberry anthocyanins were administered together with cadmium chloride to rats, it reduced cadmium accumulation in both of these organs, along with significant decreases AST and ALT activities and serum bilirubin and urea, compared to controls given cadmium only.[36]

When aminopyrine and sodium nitrite were given to rats to generate nitrosamine production, it led to liver necrosis and dystrophic changes. However, when chokeberry juice and pulp were given together with these hepatoxic substances, the liver structure was almost normal, along with decreased fat content in liver cells. Uric acid, SGOT, and SGPT were reduced in the serum due to inhibition of N-nitrosamine formation.[37]

Toxicity to the lungs from the antiarrhythmic drug amiodarone instilled in the trachea was counteracted in rats given chokeberry juice 5-10 mg/kg for 2, 5, or 10 days afterward. The cellular content and exudates in bronchoalveolar fluid and direct toxic damage to the tissues as indicated by enzyme levels were reduced to control values by both doses of the juice from day 5 onward, as was the oxidative stress and fibrosis as measured by malondialdehyde content and hydroxyproline level, respectively, by day 3. Inflammatory markers in the serum including IL-6 and IL-10 on day 3 were likewise reduced to control values by the 10 ml daily dose of the juice.[38]

Toxicity to the lungs from the antiarrhythmic
drug amiodarone instilled in the trachea was
counteracted in rats given chokeberry juice.[38]

In rats given cold-pressed chokeberry juice for 5 weeks and/or
supplemented with fructose or fat, the catalase activity in brain tissue
was signicantly decreased with consumption of the juice, compared to
no juice. Only on a high fat diet was the paraoxonase activity in the
brain tissue significantly increased, along with significantly increased
thiol groups and decreased protein carbonyl groups. This evidence
suggests that the juice helps protect the brain tissue from oxidative
stress.[39] When rats were given the juice orally in doses of 2.5, 5, or 10
mg/kg and tested for memory in a passive avoidance task, after 21 days
the 5 and 10 mg/kg doses of juice significantly and dose-dependently
improved memory retention, and after 30 days all doses were effective.
With 10 ml/kg for 30 days, the percentage of rats that reached the
learning criterion was significantly increased.[40]

In rats with endotoxin-induced uveitis, an acute intraocular
inflammation, those given a freeze-dried hydro-ethanolic chokeberry
extract in saline intravenously (i.v.) showed a dose-dependent reduction
in the number of inflammatory cells in the aqueous humor of the eye.
The 100 mg i.v. dose of polyphenol-rich extract was as effective as 10
mg i.v. prednisolone and in the aqueous humor of the eye decreased
nitric oxide, PGE_2, and TNF-α levels. The anti-inflammatory effect of
the extract was greater than equivalent amounts of only quercetin or
anthocyanins.[41]

IN VITRO

The generation of superoxide anion radicals, carbonyl groups, and
3-nitrotyrosine is significantly higher in blood platelets of 47 invasive
breast cancer patients, before and after surgery and after various phases
of chemotherapy with doxorubicin and cyclophosphamide, than in
55 healthy subjects. These oxidation markers in the platelets of breast
cancer surgery patients and chemotherapy patients, as well as in

healthy patients, were reduced significantly by exposure to a phenolic-rich extract of chokeberry. The changes in these markers, along with significant increases in reduced glutathione, indicate an alleviation of oxidative stress. This commercial extract contained 310 mg/g total phenolics: 149 mg/g phenolic acids, 111 mg/g anthocyanins, and 50 mg/g flavonoids.[42,43]

In the plasma of these 47 breast cancer patients treated with surgery and chemotherapy, the decreases of low-molecular-weight thiols, including glutathione, cysteine, and cysteinylglycine that act as free radical scavengers, were significantly improved by the commercial chokeberry phenolic-rich extract at all stages of treatment, while the elevation of the oxidant homocysteine was significantly reduced.[44] In addition, the changes in hemostatic properties, caused by the oxidative/nitrative damage in the breast cancer patients due to treatment and differing from healthy volunteers, may contribute to thrombosis in the patients. These hemostatic changes were also reduced by exposure of the plasma to the chokeberry extract.[43]

When tested in a mouse macrophage cell line, the polyphenol-rich freeze-dried hydro-ethanolic extract blocked the induction of both COX-2 and inducible nitric oxide synthase enzyme expression.[41] A similar chokeberry extract reduced lipid peroxidation induced by peroxynitrite in platelets and decreased the oxidative/nitrative stress in platelets from breast cancer patients at 50 mcg/ml.[45] Since oxidative stress can be induced by the schizophrenia drug ziprasidone, the commercial chokeberry extract rich in phenolics (phenolic acids, anthocyanins, and flavonoids) was tested on the plasma of healthy subjects after exposure to different concentrations of the drug. Lipid peroxidation induced by ziprasidone as indicated by elevated TBARS was significantly reduced by the phenolic-rich extract.[46]

When a cell culture line from a human embryonal kidney was exposed to damage from the chemotherapeutic drug cisplatin, chokeberry juice applied for 24 hours prior diminished the cytotoxicity in a concentration-dependent manner. This protection against the oxidative stress effects of the drug led to significant increase in the half maximal inhibitory concentration (IC_{50}) for cisplatin.[47] It seems unlikely that this direct tissue-protective effect would diminish the systemic therapeutic effect of cisplatin *in vivo*, since in that case the drug-treated internal tissue would not be bathed in juice.

When testing a chokeberry juice anthocyanin concentrate and fractions, the extracellular antioxidative properies were powerful for both the extract and a fraction containing both glycosides and aglycones when using the ferric reducing ability test. Also, both isolated cyanidin glycosides and the aglycone cyanidin were potent antioxidants, though fractions without these anthocyanins or this anthocyanidin were not. DNA strand breaks induced by hydrogen peroxide were significantly reduced by chokeberry juice concentrate, though not by the isolates. However, in human colon cells the generation of endogenous oxidized DNA bases was not reduced by either the concentrate, fractions, isolated anthocyanins, or cyanidin; the intracellular oxidized DNA steady state was not altered by any of these components.[48]

The ethanolic extract of the berries, its methanolic fraction and subfractions, and isolated anthocyanins were tested for DPPH radical scavenging activity. The methanolic fraction purified on Amberlite and the major anthocyanins cyanidin 3-arabinoside and cyanidin 3-galactoside and the minor cyanidin 3-glucoside had the strongest DPPH scavenging capacity, while the minor cyanidin 3-xyloside was the weakest isolate. For inhibiting 15-lipoxygenase, the 20% and 100% methanolic subfractions over Sephadex were most potent, while inhibition of alpha-glucosidase was strongest for the Amberlite methanolic fraction. The active methanolic fraction and subfractions consisted mainly of procyanidins. Cyanidin 3-arabinoside was the most potent anthocyanidin for inhibiting both of these enzymes.[49]

Examining individual anthocyanins and other polyphenolic components' antioxidant activity, it was shown that chokeberry's cyanidin-3-galactoside, cyanidin-3-arabinoside, and cyanidin-3-glucoside all have similar potency for inhibiting low-density lipoprotein (LDL) lipid peroxidation and MeLo hydroperoxide formation and in scavenging DPPH radicals. In addition, the flavonol aglycone quercetin was as, or more, potent in these same assays, while chlorogenic acid was less active for inhibiting oxidation of lipids but more effective in scavenging DPPH.[50]

CARDIOVASCULAR HEALTH AND METABOLIC SYNDROME

IN HUMANS

In a double-blind clinical study 255 mg daily of a chokeberry extract with 25% anthocyanins, 9% phenolic acids, and 50% monomeric and oligomeric procyanidins was given to 22 myocardial infarction patients who had been on the statin drugs simvastatin and atorvastatin for at least 6 months. An equal number of similar patients were given placebo. In addition, 77% of all those in the study were taking aspirin and 52% were using ACE inhibitors. Compared to those given placebo with their medications, the ones receiving the extract had significantly lowered diastolic and systolic blood pressure, C-reactive protein, IL-6, adhesion molecules, oxidized LDL, and F_2-isoprostane measurements and higher adiponectin. These changes indicated a reduction in oxidative stress and inflammatory response, suggesting a lower risk for further ischemic heart disease or "heart attack".[51]

In a study of red blood cell membranes of 25 patients with untreated hypercholesterolemia given 300 mg of the commercial phenolic-rich extract of chokeberry daily for 2 months, results were compared with a control group of 20 healthy subjects. The extract decreased erythrocyte cholesterol concentration by 22% and reduced lipid peroxidation by 40%. These results were significant after 1 and 2 months of extract supplementation. A significant increase in erythrocyte membrane fluidity was also noted after 2 months of extract use.[52]

A total of 250 ml daily of the fruit juice high in polymeric procyanidins, anthocyanins, phenolic acids, and quercetin glycosides was taken for 6 weeks by 35 hypercholesterolemic men who were not taking medications for their condition. The juice was stopped for 6 weeks, and then taken again for another 6 weeks. After the second 6-week juice intake, there were significant decreases in mean serum total cholesterol, LDL cholesterol, and triglycerides and increases in mean changes in brachial artery diameter, flow mediated dilatation, and serum nitric oxide levels, indicators of reduced cardiovascular disease risk.[53]

A similar study with 58 men with mild hypercholesterolemia used the same 250 ml daily dose of chokeberry juice for 6 weeks, then 6 weeks off, and finally another 6 weeks on. This provided a daily intake of 1065 mg total polyphenols including 734 mg polymeric procyanidins, 123 mg neochlorogenic acid, 114 mg chlorogenic acid, and 47 mg of cyanidin glycosides. There were steady significant declines in triglycerides, total cholesterol, and LDL-cholesterol over the 3 periods of the study, while high-density lipoprotein (HDL)-cholesterol significantly increased. Also found after the 18 weeks were significant decreases in glucose, homocysteine, and fibrinogen. Moreover, both systolic and diastolic blood pressures were significantly reduced after 18 weeks and between the 12th and 18th week.[54]

In a study with 38 middle-aged patients with metabolic syndrome and 14 healthy volunteer controls of equivalent age and gender ratio, 100 mg of a chokeberry extract was given 3 times daily for 2 months to those with metabolic syndrome. Each extract dose was described as containing 60 mg total polyphenols with at least 20 mg anthocyanins (65% cyanidin-3-galactoside and 29% cyanidin-3-arabinoside). Triglycerides, total cholesterol, and LDL-cholesterol were all significantly reduced in the patients after 1 and 2 months.[55]

A study examined the effects of 300 mg daily of chokeberry extract for 2 months on 25 patients with metabolic syndrome versus 22 untreated healthy control subjects. At study's end, significant reductions from baseline values were found with extract use for systolic and diastolic blood pressures, endothelin-1, total cholesterol, triglycerides, and LDL-cholesterol. Examining lipid peroxidation, the extract significantly reduced the marker TBARS and the antioxidant enzyme catalase, while significant increases were found with superoxide dismutase and glutathione peroxidase, as well as fibrinogen levels, compared to baseline.[56]

In 50 patients with metabolic syndrome, 25 who were previously non-treated received 300 mg daily of chokeberry extract (with 60 mg total polyphenols, 20 mg anthocyanins) for 2 months, while 25 active controls were taking an angiotensin I-converting enzyme (ACE) inhibitor and hypolipemic medication, and an additional 20 healthy controls had no intervention. Those receiving the extract had significant reductions in total cholesterol, LDL, systolic blood pressure (SBP), and ACE activity after 1 and 2 months. However, the LDL, SBP, and ACE activity values were still significantly higher than healthy controls, as was the SBP of conventionally-treated controls.[57]

IN ANIMALS

Chokeberry juice high in phenolics (709 mg/100 ml) including anthocyanins (107 mg/100 ml) was fed at 5, 10, or 20 ml/kg b.w. for 30 days to rats on a control diet or on a control diet plus 4% cholesterol. There were no changes in plasma lipids with the juice for rats on the control diet. Those consuming 4% cholesterol and juice had significantly reduced elevations in total cholesterol and LDL-cholesterol at all dosages and triglycerides at the 20 ml/kg dose, compared to diet alone. HDL-cholesterol and liver or aorta histology were not significantly altered by the diets or the juice.[58]

Assessing effects on metabolic syndrome disposition in rats with induced hyperlipidemia, oxidative stress, and glucose intolerance from streptozotocin and a high-fructose diet, a polyphenol-rich (714 mg/g with 56.6% anthocyanins) extract of chokeberry as 0.2% of the diet lowered cholesterol and improved antioxidant status, including normalizing lipid peroxidation in liver, kidneys, and lungs. It also showed hypoglycemic activity, decreasing sucrase and maltase activity and increasing lactase activity in the intestinal mucosa. Chokeberry is seen as a promising means of helping avoid metabolic syndrome and its complications.[59]

To induce insulin resistance, rats were fed a fructose-rich diet for 6 weeks with or without a spray-dried chokeberry extract, made from frozen berries with 60% ethanol and containing at least 10% anthocyanins, that was added to the drinking water at 100 or 200 mg/kg b.w. daily. Both doses significantly reduced weight gain and blood glucose, cholesterol, LDL-cholesterol, and triglycerides. In addition, the extract inhibited the inflammatory cytokines TNF-α and IL-6, while significantly elevating HDL-cholesterol adiponectin levels in the plasma, compared to controls. These effects were credited to changes in gene expression.[60]

In apolipoprotein E knockout mice fed a diet with 15% fat and 0.2% cholesterol, those that also received 0.05% of a spray-dried chokeberry ethanolic extract rich in polyphenols (131.6 mg/g anthocyanins, 100.6 mg/g chlorogenic/neochlorogenic acids, and 10.2 mg/g quercetin and its glycosides) had 12% less plasma total cholesterol than controls. Plasma catalase and paraoxonase activities were increased significantly in the mice receiving the 0.05% extract diet, along with increased liver glutathione peroxidase activity. While the plasma and liver antioxidant function increased, the plasma cholesterol decreased independent of liver gene expression associated with cholesterol metabolism.[61]

In rats with hypertension induced by L-NG-nitroarginine methyl ester (L-NAME), those given 0.05 g/kg body weight of an ethanolic extract of dried ripe chokeberries every other day with L-NAME for 8 weeks had significantlyly lower blood pressure values compared to L-NAME-only rats, along with significantly higher total antioxidant capacity. The extract contained 24.9 mg/g total phenolics and 4.46 mcmoles/g anthocyanins; phenolics identified specifically included chlorogenic acid, rutin, hyperoside, quercetin, and kuromanin. Serum glutathione peroxidase activity was significantly higher in rats receiving the extract, while reduced glutathione content was normalized and the lipid peroxidation marker malondialdehyde was reduced considerably.[62]

In Vitro

For inhibition of angiotensin I-converting enzyme (ACE), the IC_{50} of a chokeberry extract was 155.4 mcg/ml, compared to 0.52 mcg/ml for the ACE inhibitor drug captopril.[57] ACE inhibitors are used from reducing blood pressure in hypertensive patients.

An anthocyanin-rich chokeberry extract was tested on coronary arterial rings from pigs in isometric force studies. The extract produced dose- and endothelium-dependent vasorelaxation. At a concentration of 0.05 mg/L total anthocyanins, the greatest protection was shown against reactive oxygen species (ROS)-induced loss of relaxation produced by the compound A23187. Extract concentrations lower than necessary to alter the vascular tone still protect the coronary arteries from ROS without altering relaxation to nitric oxide, suggesting it could have significant benefits in vascular disease.[63]

Human aortic endothelial cell treated with 50 mcg/ml of chokeberry fruit extract prior to TNF-α exposure significantly inhibited the expression of ICAM-1 and VCAM-1, decreased NF-κB activation, and reduced intracellular ROS production. In so doing, it showed anti-inflammatory effects that could provide cardioprotective benefits.[64]

The impact of chokebrry extract on Caco-2 intestinal mucosal cells showed this polyphenol-rich preparation regulates gene expression associated with cholesterol absorption and lipid metabolism. Apical cholesterol uptake was significantly decreased, while mRNA was induced that mediates apical cholesterol efflux. The extract significantly increased the mRNA and protein levels of low-density lipoprotein (LDL) receptor, as well as cellular LDL uptake. This effects likely contribute to hypolipidemic activity of chokeberry extracts.[65]

COAGULATION

IN HUMANS

In a study of blood clotting with 38 patients with metabolic syndrome and 14 matched healthy volunteer controls, 300 mg of a chokeberry extract containing 180 mg total polyphenols was given daily to the patients for 2 months. At baseline and continuing for 2 months, when platelet-rich plasma was separated and tested *ex vivo*, the fibrinogen was significantly higher in the plasma from metabolic syndrome patients than in controls; however, the potential for clotting and fibrinolysis was reduced significantly from baseline after 1 month to control levels. In addition, after 1 month the maximal aggregation induced by ADP was significantly decreased in patients compared to baseline, along with significantly reductions in maximum clotting and overall potential for coagulation to match control values. After 2 months the potential for clotting remained significantly decreased, while the thrombin generation time was significantly increased. Thus, hemostatic parameters improved in metabolic syndrome patients. No significant changes were seen with control subjects.[55]

IN VITRO

A commercial Polish chokeberry extract, containing about 60% total phenolics and at least 20% anthocyanins, at concentrations between 5-100 mcg/ml significantly and dose-dependently reduced aggregation of platelets both from 15 patients with cardiovascular risks (hypertension, hypercholesterolemia, smoking, diabetes) and from 15 healthy controls. This occurred whether platelet aggregation was induced by collagen or thrombin and independently of nitric oxide release by platelets. A reduction in superoxide production in those with cardiovascular risks was not associated with the anti-aggregatory effects.[66]

Using the same chokeberry extract, platelet aggregation inhibition induced by human umbilical vein endothelial cells on ADP-activated platelets from 16 healthy men and women was shown to be significantly enhanced at the low concentration of 5 mcg/ml.[67] Spontaneous and ADP-activated platelet adhesion was also reduced by aronia extract at 10-100 mcg/ml. The extract also significantly inhibited the amidolytic activity of both thrombin and plasmin at these concentrations.[68]

When fresh plasma and human thrombin were incubated together with 5 mcg/ml of the same commercial extract of chokeberry, the clotting time was significantly prolonged in a dose-dependent manner, and the fibrin polymerization maximal velocity in human plasma was significantly decreased. The extract was analyzed and shown to contain 478 mg/g total phenolics, including 135 mg/g total hydroxycinnamic acids, 94 mg/g each of total anthocyanins and total flavanols, and 24 mg/g total flavonols.[69]

A follow-up study with this same extract showed that in the 0.5-50 mcg/ml range it both dose-dependently and significantly inhibited thrombin-induced fibrinogen polymerization and platelet aggregation, while also stabilizing formation of fibrin. Of individual phenolic components that were tested for their effect on the amidolytic activity of thrombin, the aglycone cyanidin had the lowest inhibitory concentration, 20 time more potent than cyanidin 3-glucoside and almost twice as potent as quercetin. Inhibiting thrombin is a major trend in pharmacotherapy to prevent thrombotic states, so the potential for identifying an effective orally-bioavailable polyphenolic alternative to vitamin K antagonists like warfarin in enticing.[70]

High concentrations of homocysteine in its reduced (0.1 mM) and its most reactive form (1 mcM) induce oxidative stress and fibrinogen polymerization in plasma, but chokeberry extract at 5.0 mcg/ml was shown to reduce these biotoxicity actions, similar to resveratrol. This suggests the extract may be protective against thrombosis in hyperhomocysteinemia.[71] When peroxynitrite was added to plasma it led to nitrative damage to the fibrinogen, but chokeberry extract added at 0.5-50 mcg/ml to the fibrinogen 10 minutes prior protected against this.[72]

CHEMOPREVENTIVE POTENTIAL OF CHOKEBERRY DERIVATIVES

IN ANIMALS

In a test of mice exposed to cigarette smoke daily from birth to 4 months of age, some were also given chokeberry aqueous extract in the only source of drinking water for 7 months beginning at weaning. Those mice without the extract developed weight loss, lung alterations including adenomas and emphasema, cytogenetical damage to red blood cells, liver parenthymal degeneration, and bladder epithelial hyperplasia. Mice consuming the extract showed inhibition of all of these effects, except for bladder epithelial hyperplasia. Due to the extensive protection from a complex toxin, the outcome suggests a multitude of active components and mechanisms.[73]

An anthocyanin-rich extract of Indiana chokeberries was given for 14 weeks to rats treated with the colon carcinogen azoxymethan and compared to controls. The rats given the extract consumed about 26 mg/kg of anthocyanins and 111 mg/kg total phenolics per day. Total and large aberrant crypt foci were reduced significantly by the extract. Colon cellular proliferation was decreased by the extract diet. High levels of fecal anthocyanins were detected, along with increased fecal mass and moisture and a reduction of fecal bile acids, compared to controls. These findings suggest multiple protective effects of the anthocyanins against colon carcinogenesis.[25]

Chokeberry juice was given to rats by gavage at 8 ml/kg b.w. for 28 days; on day 27, the carcinogen N-nitrosodiethylamine (NDEA) was injected intraperitoneally (i.p.) into these and into control rats. After NDEA exposure the rats that had consumed the juice for 4 weeks had partial protection from its toxicity, as the elevations of sorbitol dehydrogenase (SDH), gamma glutamyl transferase (GGT), bilirubin, and creatinin were significantly less than mice receiving only NDEA. However, possibly due to the liver carcinogen NDEA having the same effects on CYP1A1 and CYP1A2, along with NDEA decreasing the activity of CYP2E1 and enhancing CYP2B and NAD(P)H:quinone oxidoreductase-1 (NQO1) activity, the juice significantly increased DNA damage caused by NDEA.[74] This finding stands in contrast to the rest of the studies that show anticancer potential.

Rats that were also given 8 ml/kg chokeberry juice for 28 days by gavage were in this case administered the liver and mammary gland carcinogen 7,12-dimethylbenz[a]anthracen (DMBA) i.p. on the day 27. Juice consumption again provided partial protection from liver toxicity, as the elevations by DMBA of SDH, GGT, and alanine aminotransferase (ALT), along with bilirubin, creatinine, and blood urea nitrogen (BUN) were significantly reduced. The juice reduced activity of CYP1A1 and CYP1A2 and NQO1 in the liver, but not in mammary glands. These isoenzymes are involved in DMBA metabolic conversion, but the juce had no effect on DMBA-induced DNA damage in blood cells. Thus, chokeberry effects on carcinogen metabolism depend on the carcinogen and are tissue specific.[75]

In Vitro

An anthocyanin-rich extract of chokeberry induced apoptosis in human pancreatic cancer cells at a concentration of 1 mcg/ml such that it also increased the cytotoxicity of the chemotherapy agent gemcitabine, when used in combination against this cell line AsPC-1 *in vitro*.[76] A glioblastoma cell line (U373) treated for 48 hours with chokeberry extract or curcumin found IC_{50} values of 200 and 15 mcg/ml, respectively. Chokeberry extract caused cell line necrosis, while curcumin induces apoptosis. Both downregulated gene expression for matrix metalloproteinases (MMP)-2, -14, -16, and -17. These effects both demonstrate anticancer potential.[77]

In human HT-29 colon cancer cell cultures, an anthocyanin-rich extract of chokeberry fruit inhibited growth by 60%, with a blockage at both cell cycle G1/G0 and G2/M phases. This coincided with altered gene expression, including decreased COX-2 and cyclin A and B gene expression. Normal colon cells were not similarly effected, with <10% growth inhibition at the highest concentration of 50 mcg/ml.[78]

Human colon carcinoma Caco-2 cells exposed 2 hours daily for 4 days to chokeberry juice subjected to gastric and pancreatic digestion *in vitro* led to G2/M cell cycle arrest. In conjunction the tumor suppressor carcinoembryonic antigen-related cell adhesion molecule 1 (CEACAM1) was up-regulated at both the mRNA and protein levels; its expression is typically reduced in early carcinomas and adenomas.[79]

Among 35 beverages tested for the influence on estradiol sulfation in Caco-2 cells, aronia juice was the second strongest inhibitor after coffee. These drinks strongly inhibited sulfotransferase activity on estrogen in these human colon cancer cells. Since colon cancer incidence in women is reportedly reduced in those who drink coffee, there may be a relationship between colon cancer and sulfotransferase activity.[10]

Good correlation was shown between total procyanidin and anthocyanin content of chokeberry extract and its antioxidant activity. The anthocyanin fraction of a chokeberry extract was found to inhibit proliferation of HeLa human cervical tumor cells. The anthocyanins also increased intracellular reactive oxygen species generation after 48 hours, a possible mechanism for the antiproliferative effect.[80]

Crude extracts with 70% aqueous acetone were made from Illinois wild and European cultivated chokeberries and compared, along with 6 fractions and 22 subfractions, for effects on L1210 leukemia cells. A fraction of the wild berries at 50 mcg/ml inhibited the leukemia cell activity by >95%, while a similar subfraction from the cultivated berries at 25 mcg/ml showed a >90% inhibition. All of the fractions from the wild berries acted as topoisomerase inhibitors.[16]

In the lymphoblastic leukemia Jurkat cell line, chokeberry juice from Germany with 7.15 g/L polyphenols inhibited cell proliferation. Cell cycle arrest occurred in the G_2/M phase, the juice inducing apoptosis associated with upregulation of active caspase 3 and tumor suppressor p73. The juice also increased formation of reactive oxygen species to produce a sustained intracellular pro-oxidant effect. (Similar effects have been shown with resveratrol, EGCG, and curcumin.) Fractionation identified anticancer activity in association primarily with chlorogenic acids, some cyanidin glycosides, and quercetin derivatives. The juice also induced apoptosis in other human lymphoblastic leukemia cells including HSB-2, Molt-4, and CCRF-CEM lines and in human primary lymphoblastic leukemia cells, but not in normal primary T-lymphocytes.[81]

A significant reduction in mutagenic changes has been shown with chokeberry fruit anthocyanins. Sister chromatid exchanges induced by the carcinogen benzo(a)pyrene in human lymphocytes cultures were significantly decreased by the anthocyanins. The reduction of sister chromatid exchanges from exposure to mitomycin C was not as great, but was noticeable. This effect was thought to be due to free radical scavenging and inhibition of enzymes that activate these promutagens.[82]

CHOKEBERRY AND INFECTIONS

IN HUMANS

In a crossover intervention for prevention of urinary tract infection (UTI), residents in 6 nursing homes were given placebo for 80 days and then chokeberry juice for 65 days (group A; 110 residents in 4 nursing homes) or the juice for 40 days and placebo for 30 days (group B; 126 residents in 2 nursing homes). Periods of 3 months observation were undertaken before and after the 2 consecutive periods of receiving placebo or juice. The total phenolic content including anthocyanins, chlorgenic acids, and B-type procyanidins in the 156 ml daily juice intake by group A was 1115 mg, while the 89 ml juice daily consumed by group B contained 636 mg phenolics. During the period of juice consumption, there was no reduction in antibiotic use or UTI frequency, but in the subsequent

3-month period the incidence of UTIs was reduced in group A by 55% and in group B by 38%.[83]⟨◈⟩

In Animals

Mice, exposed intranasally to 5 times the 50% mouse lethal dose of influenza virus strain rPR8-GFP, were untreated or treated orally twice daily for 3 days with either 1 mg/kg of the antiviral drug oseltamivir or chokeberry alcoholic extract, or i.p. with the chokeberry components ellagic acid or myricetin. The viral expressions in the lung tissue were reduced more than 50% by the chokeberry extract, ellagic acid, and myricetin, compared to non-treated mice, and viral replication was reduced 15-30%, while morbidity was likewise reduced. All untreated mice died within 10 days, whereas those on oseltamivir all survived 14 days, and mice receiving chokeberry extract, ellagic acid, and myricetin had 14-day survival rates of 50%, 50%, and 37.5%, respectively.[84]

> The viral expressions in the lung tissue were reduced more than 50% by the chokeberry extract, ellagic acid, and myricetin, compared to non-treated mice. [84]

In Vitro

When tested against seasonal influenza viruses (H1/K09, H3/PE16, B/BR60), oseltamivir-resistant strain (H1/K2785), and H5N1 influenza virus (HPAI rH5/IS06), chokeberry ethanolic extract showed cross-reactive efficacy with 0.0625-0.5 mg mixed in 200 mcL of media; 0.125 mg had >60% efficacy against all viruses tested. Higher concentrations were needed for H5 and human B subtypes, and increased concentrations in general were more effective. Of the 7 polyphenolic constituents tested, 4 restrained H1/K09 viral replication: ellagic acid, gallic acid, myricetin, and quercetin.[84]

In a test of chokeberry extracts, subfractions, and compounds for inhibiting *Escherichia coli* and *Bacillus cereus* and preventing biofilm formation, no bacterial inhibition was detected. Still, an anti-biofilm activity was shown against *B. cereus* strain 407 most strongly by the 50% ethanolic extract, but also a 50 ℃ water extract, the anthocyanin cyanidin-3-xyloside, neochlorogenic acid, procyanidins B2, B5, and C1, and a polymeric procyanidin fraction Seph g. On the other hand, epicatechin and 3 anthocyanins (cyanidin-3-galactoside, -glucoside, and -arabinoside) actually increased *B. cereus* biofilm growth. Anti-biofilm activity against *E. coli* strain JM109 was shown with the 50% ethanolic extract, both the 50 ℃ and 100 ℃ water extracts, dichloromethane extract, cyanidin-3-xyloside, and especially epicatechin. In this case, the procyanidin monomers, Seph G, and the other 3 anthocyanins increased *E. coli* biofilm.[85]

In tests on inhibiting the nitric oxide (NO) production in lipopolysaccharide-induced macrophages, procyanidins B2, B5, and C1 plus proanthocyanidin-rich fractions with degree of polymerization (PD) of 7 and 34 were active. All except the fraction with PD 34 were inhibitory to NO without impacting cell viability, demonstrating an anti-inflammatory effect. These same procyanidins and proanthocyanidin fractions, plus the aglycone cyanidin, also showed strong complement-fixing activities.[86]

POTENTIAL ALTERATIONS IN DRUG METABOLISM

IN HUMANS

A human case report described, after a fourth cycle of trabectedin as second-line chemotherapy, a man with liposarcoma who suddenly developed weakness and diffuse muscle pain. This occurred only after taking a chokeberry preparation during the last course of trabectin and the following 2 weeks. Along with increased serum levels of myoglobin, creatinine phosphokinase, and lactate dehydrogenase, there was evidence of pancytopenia and a large increase in liver enzymes. After stopping the chokeberry extract, the markers of myolysis slowly returned to normal and muscle strength progressively recovered. The evidence indicated that it was probable the adverse event was an interaction of trabectedin and chokeberry, likely through inhibition of CYP3A4, though this conclusion is speculative.[87]

It was probable the adverse event was an interaction of trabectedin and chokeberry.[87]

In Animals

Chokeberry juice was given to rats by gavage at 8 ml/kg body weight for 28 days. Chokeberry decreased activities of hepatic cytochrome P450 (CYP) 1A1 and CYP1A2 and increased CYP2B. Phase II metabolic enzymes glutathione-S-transferase and quinone reductase were both increased by the juice in the liver,[74,75] but not in mammary glands.[75]

In Vitro

Of 27 compounds isolated and identified from the ethyl acetate-soluble extract of chokeberry, the 3 that were shown to double phase II quinone reductase activity in micromolar amounts were quercetin at 3.1 mcM, protocatechuic acid at 4.3 mcM, and neochlorogenic acid methyl ester at 6.7 mcM.[88]

Using the sedative drug midazolam as a substrate demonstrated that cyanidin-3-arabinoside is a more potent CYP3A4 inhibitor than the more abundant cyanidin-3-galactoside and the minor cyanidin-3-glucoside. Procyanidin B5 is likewise a stronger inhibitor than its isomeric procyanidin B2. Proanthocyanidin fraction CYP3A4 inhibitory activity is based on the degree of polymerization.[89]

Summary

The potent antioxidant effect from the polyphenolic compounds in chokeberry, especially its anthocyanins, has been shown to protect tissues from damage due to toxins and various oxidizing agents. The impact on endothelial function has demonstrated benefits in clinical studies for those with cardiovascular disease and those at risk. Research evidence is particularly supportive of those who suffer with metabolic syndrome, that is, those who are have excessive abdominal fat with hyperlipidemia and/or diabetes risk and/or high blood pressure, along with underlying oxidative stress and low-grade inflammation.

Common dosage forms including juice and extracts can readily provide the effective anthocyanin dosage for this condition. To help avoid vascular obstruction by blood clots, the reduction of coagulation propensities by thrombin inhibition is very attractive as a potential alternative to vitamin K antagonists known for the having a poor safety profile. Counteracting changes that make tissues susceptible to cancer or insidious degenerative diseases suggests chokeberry is a viable means of reducing chronic disease risk.

More limited evidence suggests possible benefits of chokeberry in cases of urinary tract infection and influenza. Similarly, preclinical research and a human case report also suggest potential inhibition of some drug metabolism; however, such limited evidence is an inadequate basis on which to draw clinical conclusions. Preclinical research showing enhancement of phase II elimination of certain metabolic byproducts likewise renders this as a possibility. As this once relatively inaccessible berry becomes more widespread through commercial cultivation and utilization and is examined in good quality human studies and clinical trials, its value and limitation will be revealed. Chokeberry's growing availability will provide another fruitful opportunity for those who desire the protection against oxidative stress that can be gained from this polyphenol-rich source and its dietary and supplemental preparations.

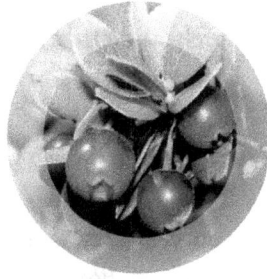

FIVE

A PERSPECTIVE ON BERRY RESEARCH AND HEALTH

DUE TO THEIR RADICAL-SCAVENGING, ANTIOXIDANT, AND ANTI-INFLAMMATORY ACTIVITIES, THE WIDE VARIETIES OF BIOACTIVE POLYPHENOLICS INCLUDING ANTHOCYANINS AND OTHER FLAVONOIDS, PHENOLIC ACIDS, STILBENES, AND PROANTHOCYANIDINS IN BERRIES AND OTHER FRUITS, AS WELL AS IN VEGETABLES, HERBS, AND SPICES, ARE VITALLY NECESSARY FOR PROTECTING AND MAINTAINING OPTIMAL HEALTH. IN A WORLD WHERE EXPOSURE TO DAMAGING SYNTHETIC CHEMICAL COMPOUNDS IS AN INESCAPABLE REALITY, REDUCING THE IMPACT OF INSIDIOUSLY TOXIC SUBSTANCES IS NECESSARY FOR AVOIDING CELLULAR AND TISSUE OXIDATIVE STRESS AND PRO-INFLAMMATORY STATES THAT CAN PREDISPOSE PEOPLE TO CHRONIC DISEASES.

In the past, fresh berries were only available seasonally. Widespread cultivation, modern processing technologies, and efficient transportation has made access to some fresh berries possible much of the year, while many berries are available all year in fresh-frozen form. The phytochemical compositions of berry products can be highly variable depending on differences in cultivars, geographic origins, harvesting, processing, and storage. Combining several types of products, especially if one source is canned goods, is more likely to provide meaningful amounts of the broad spectrum of protective nutrient and non-nutritive agents.

An important aspect of a healthy diet is to enjoy a variety of fresh garden and orchard foods, including fresh and/or frozen berries. Obtaining, preparing, and safely and effectively preserving fresh berries can be challenging, but relying only on consumption of commercially processed preparations is not optimal. To supplement occasional or even frequent intake of fresh or frozen berries, freeze-dried concentrated berry powders or extracts can help assure a steady intake on a daily basis. These more concentrated sources offer simple means of maintaining regular exposure for long-term use. For convenience of consumption, canned products including juices have their place as available options as well.

Juices from cranberry and aronia, like their concentrated extracts, have been shown to benefit or prevent some chronic conditions. Even frozen berry juice concentrates added to smoothies or sparkling water provide add value to these beverages. However, any type of juice or extract contains only a portion of the overall value from the berry. In general, overall juice consumption should be limited to moderate amounts (8-12 oz. daily) because of the sugar content and lack of fiber. Juice from sources like cranberries that are low in sugar can be unpalatable in its pure natural form. Mixing this sour juice with sugars or combining it with sweet juices like those made from grapes or pears helps solve the taste issue but introduces the sugar problem. Artificial sweeteners, intended to improve the flavor and to help avoid over-consumption of sugars, are unnatural synthetic chemicals. Recent development of extractives from the stevia plant has made available safe, non-caloric sweetening agents from a natural source.

> In general, overall juice consumption should be limited to moderate amounts (8-12 oz. daily) because of the sugar content and lack of fiber.

Air-dried berries provide antioxidant activity and good fiber, but are still relatively high in sugars and have lost much of the antioxidant value available in fresh or frozen berries. Drawbacks such as nutrient loss and excessive sugar apply even more to other highly processed and sweetened products, such as preserves, jams, and jellies. These are best suited for occassional use in small amounts by individuals with normal sugar metabolism. Berry pies and cobblers can be nutritious desserts, but, when excessively sweetened, are likewise not appropriate as part of the regular diet. Over-consumption of sugars is one of the major factors contributing to many of the chronic conditions that currently plague humanity, especially obesity and type 2 diabetes. The different forms of foods and beverages prepared from berries provide some delectable choices that can make their consumption more enjoyable, but the less sugars ingested, the healthier the outcome.

⊗ Though berries in general share many of the same benefits, since as a group they are more concentrated in anthocyanins than most other fruit, each kind of berry offers specific advantages that are greater than found in other sources. Blueberries have become known for helping protect the brain from neurodegenerative disorders, especially those involving memory. As populations age, this becomes a critical concern for maintaining self-reliance and independence. Cranberry juice is an established means of decreasing urinary tract infections but has now been recognized for reducing markers indicative of cardiovascular disease. Freeze-dried black raspberries hold promise as a means of helping prevent cancers of the digestive tract by direct local exposure. Finally, chokeberry may be the berry best suited for lowering risk factors involved with cardiovascular and coagulation risks. ⊗

All these berries are known for their high potential for reducing cellular oxidative stress, the underlying condition that contributes to many chronic disease conditions. Noteworthy among these modern epidemics is the ever-expanding metabolic syndrome (that includes abdominal obesity, hyperlipidemia, high blood pressure, and/or glucose intolerance); all four of these berries have shown evidence of helping ameliorate this condition. The reduction of carcinogenicity of chemical substances and radiation is another potential advantage derived from these four berries. Protection against foreign chemical compounds in general through enhanced metabolic processing in the liver appears to be part of the mechanism for black raspberry and chokeberry. Reducing susceptibility to infection is potentially an additional berry benefit, while diminishing the expression of low-grade inflammation with these berries is another contributing factor to promoting overall long-term health.

Ingesting delicious food preparations and good quality dietary supplement products that provide essential and adjunctive nutritional benefits is an enjoyable and immanently practical means of addressing major health concerns that plague our modern world. Berries have been shown scientifically to be helpful for preventing or reducing oxidative and/or inflammatory features underlying many common diseases. The means for addressing many of these contemporary ills lies within our grasp, when made available on our tables in the form of traditional foods, especially those from plants. Berries, like other fruits and vegetables, herbs, and spices, are desirable for their distinctive flavors and attractive colorful appearances. Now, more than ever, they all need to be appreciated, eaten, enjoyed, and advocated for their life-enhancing and health-ensuring compositions of savory and potent bioactive content.

APPENDIX: ADVANTAGES AND LIMITATIONS OF DIFFERENT FORMS AND PREPARATIONS

FRESH BERRIES

Throughout the ages, fresh berries have been the preferred form for consumption. This most happily occurs while picking them from the bush or bramble, usually while collecting more for later enjoyment at home. One of my most pleasurable childhood memories is of sitting in the shade of the branches of a mulberry tree on a hot summer day with the sweet juice filling my mouth and staining my fingers purple. A little dust on these luscious gems did not diminish the experience in the least. Such times spent in nature and enjoying its bounty and goodness are indelibly imprinted on my psyche.

Fresh berries, washed and preferably organic, are certainly a great way to enjoy these fruit, and the optimal way to obtain the full nutritional value. The juiciness of fresh fruit and berries allows the flavor and nutrients to be immediately released with a little chewing, even delivering health benefits to the mouth and esophagus. Unsurprisingly, consumption of fruit is associated with reduced cancer risk in these organs and the throat, and even in the larynx. The berry water itself, both that which is filtered through the roots plus the new water unique to that plant as a product of its photosynthesis, is an essential component in sustaining the complex phytochemical integrity that makes fresh berries tantalizing and in delivering nourishment directly to those tissues that come in immediate contact with the juice.

One advantage of fresh berries is their wide applicability, when eaten alone from the hand, added on top of cooked or cold cereal, baked in breads, or used to color salads. They enhance the flavor of otherwise bland foods, mixed in live plain yogurt for breakfast or with a little real vanilla ice cream as a treat. (The higher the ratio of berries to ice cream, the better it is.) These are ingredients that children love, so it is good to doctor-up less tasty dishes with a child's favorite berries. They help bring back pleasant memories of better days for the ailing elderly as well.

Some berries may be too sour to enjoy fresh or alone. I remember my mother adding sour wild gooseberries to her mulberry pies to enhance the flavors of both. Fresh berries mix well with each other and with other fresh fruit, expanding the culinary possibilities as good combinations harmonize flavors and complement nutrients. Consequently, varying fruit salads can provide different enjoyable dishes without one becoming tired of the same flavors. However, many fresh berries have a very limited shelf life, especially when obtained in such abundance that adequate refrigeration is unavailable, so preserving berries for longer use is also necessary.

Means of traditional home preservation typically included air-drying or canning whole berries, canning preserves and jams, or extracting the juice for making wine and jellies. Using heat and sugar or alcohol as means of preserving delicious berry flavors has been a common but less than optimal way of retaining some of the nutrient richness. Therefore, with the exception of fresh juice or canning non-sweetened whole berries in berry juice, air-drying berries may preferable in a nutritional sense to these other forms of preservation.

While the above processes will all be briefly described below, a couple of modern means that are the most preferable ways of preserving berries will be highlighted first. Foremost of these, the advent of freezing berries has made seasonal fruit available all year while retaining the components in the fresh berry, including its water medium. Freezing thereby optimally retains the phytochemical proportions and bioactivity associated with fresh "living" berries after storage. The second method utilizes freezing prior to vacuum drying, providing a dry powder that contains the components found in the fresh berry by freeze-drying.

FROZEN BERRIES

Like drying, freezing essentially "kills" the berry. In this case the cell membranes are ruptured by the expanding ice as the intracellular water freezes. By keeping the nutrients in suspension, it nonetheless mixes the compartmentalized nutrients and enzymes, so that when the frozen berries thaw the inner berry has largely been "juiced", while containing all of the original matrix elements including fiber. However, enzymes become active when released and lead to chemical conversions of some compounds that can alter flavor. Also, the turgidity that the intact cellular membranes provide for the fresh berry is lost, so the frozen-then-thawed berry become softened.

The great advantage of freezing is that it allows the storage of berries in their whole, entire state for a prolonged period. Nutrient content is reduced over time, based on the storage temperature and the duration of storage. Therefore, berries should not be stored indefinately in home freezers but should be consumed before the next fruiting season when fresh berries become available. The thawed berries can be consumed in many of the same ways as fresh berries, though leakage of juice and potential staining can obviously be an issue. Dishes, bowls, and spoons become a necessity, whereas they serve as suitable social options with fresh berries in situations where eating with ones fingers may be perceived as gauche.

FREEZE-DRIED BERRIES

Freeze-drying, known also by the technical term lyophilization, was developed during World War II to ship blood serum from America to Europe; it was then also applied to preserving penicillin. Freeze-drying grew in utilization in the latter half of the twentieth century in both pharmaceutical applications and the food and beverage industries. Lyophilization uses the process of sublimation to remove water from substance by first freezing the substance, and then lowering the pressure in a partial vacuum which causes the ice to transform directly to water vapor. To complete the drying, the temperature is slowly raised in the vacuum dryer to above freezing. This process causes the rapid removal of water with heating and without allowing a liquid phase in which enzymatic transformations can occur. Since it is a physical and not a chemical process, it does not introduce new compounds into the freeze-dried material, but maintains the chemical integrity of the material almost in its entirely.

Freeze-dried berries maintain their original appearance when kept whole, unlike other dried berries. They absorb water better due to internal cell rupture, so they reconstitute more rapidly and by appearance more completely. Freeze-dried berries are often added to breakfast cereals, whether prepared hot or cold, and make a wonderful addition to trail mixes and other dry snacks. Another advantage of freeze-dried berries is the extensive shelf-life, if they are kept dry and away from light in opaque sealed containers or resealable foil bags. As with any form, the lower the temperature used for storage, the longer the preservation of the original phytochemical contents, so refrigeration or frozen storage of freeze-dried berries further extends the shelf life. When kept this way, the berry components are most stable for long-term storage.

Yet, they may be even better in some regards when they are ground to powder and used in moist foods like yogurt or added to smoothies or apple sauce. The reason for this is the increase in surface area of the particles of powder allows for even more rapid and complete hydration, which then helps enhance the digestion and absorption of the nutrients contained in the dried berry, something not as achievable with gummy "dried" berries or fruit like raisins or prunes. If the berries are powdered, they require a desiccant in opaque or brown glass bottles to absorb moisture.

On a further note, powdering freeze-dried berries releases access to potent phytochemicals in seeds that would otherwise pass undigested through the gut, if the berries where eaten fresh and chewed normally. In particular, berries in the Rosacea family including strawberries, raspberries, and blackberries contain high amounts of the antioxidant ellagic acid in their seeds, more even than in any other part of the berry or plant. These typically pass whole through the intestines, since vigorous chewing is required to crack through the seed shell and mash them flat. Even then, the seeds remain largely intact, making it difficult to absorb ellagic acid. So, in the regard, freeze-drying these berries may in some ways exceed the benefits from the fresh fruit due to the enhanced bioavailability of ellagic acid and its derivatives.

Powdering the freeze-dried berries makes them easier to add, alone or in combinations, to a liquid preparation for consumption. However, the dissolution of the freeze-dried berry powder does not occur instantaneously like many granulated "instant drinks" or freeze-dried juice, since the whole berry powder contains all of the berry fiber but no additives, so the powder retains some degree of cohesion. To effectively address this, either a mechanical stirrer or blender can be used. Otherwise, if small lumps have formed in the powder container, pressing them against the side of the container with a fork readily breaks the lumps.

Adding a spoonful of freeze-dried berry powder straight into water or juice can cause a clump to form on the surface, with powder in the middle of the clump still dry. A simple and quite effective method to address this is to use a closed bottle, jar, or container as a shaker. After adding the freeze-dried powder to water, juice, or other fluid in the bottle or jar, replace the cap or lid firmly and manually shake the container 5 or 10 times. The impact of the powder and fluid on the sides of the bottle or jar disperses the powder into the liquid. After drinking the mixture from the container, some wet whole-berry powder will have adhered to the sides and bottom. By adding a little water or juice and reshaking, this powder readily dislodges into solution and can then be consumed.

FRESH AND FREEZE-DRIED BERRY JUICE

After fresh, fresh frozen, and fresh freeze-dried berries, probably the next best form of deriving the most goodness from berries would be consuming small amounts of the fresh juice. I note small amounts, since juicing vastly reduces the bulk such that a small amount of juice represents a large serving of berries. (How much depends upon the type of berry, its initial fluid content, and the efficiency of extracting the juice.) The value is in its freshness, and in the quality of the original berry water in the fresh juice, as opposed to the filtered tap water used to reconstitute commercial "100% juice" from concentrates.

Unfortunately, once its made the juice can begin to rapidly deteriorate due to the activation of enzymes caused by cellular wall and membrane rupture in the juicing process. This mixing leads to relatively rapid conversions of compounds in the berries that can alter the taste and effects. Refrigeration helps to slow these enzymatic breakdowns, but the best means of stopping this from occurring is to freeze-dry the fresh juice. This takes the phytochemical content including enzymes out of solution, so the enzymatic reactions cannot occur while in the dried state. The advantage of freeze-dried juice over freeze-dried berries is the relatively greater ease of dissolution of the dried juice into water or other solution compared to the dried and powdered whole berry. On the other hand, much of the beneficial nutrient content of the berry is lost in the process of juicing, so if it is to then be freeze-dried it results in an inferior quality, though more convenient, product.

Disadvantages to juice include the loss of fiber, but not only fiber. Many important phytochemicals, including the anthocyanin pigments that function as potent antioxidants, are bound to the fiber and lost with it. In the case of cranberry juice, the powerful triterpene component ursolic acid is lost in the pomace, the fibrous berry residue left behind. Being a liquid form, juice is rapidly absorbed and bioavailable, so it quickly raises blood levels of its absorbed components which are then more rapidly excreted. This provides higher concentrations of phytochemicals in the urine. By comparison, when the whole fruit or berry is consumed with its fiber, not only are all the phytochemicals available, but they transit the intestinal tract for a longer period of time. This allows for more gradual absorption, with lower blood levels that are maintained over a longer period of time, and lower urinary concentration. In addition, the lining of the distal intestinal tract receives exposure to these phytochemicals as they travel further throught the digestive tract. So, the forms of berry preparations not only help determine the contents, but also the effects of that content on different parts of the body.

CANNED BERRIES AND JUICE

The disadvantage of canning berries lies in the fact that preservation by canning involves using heat which is necessary to destroy microorgainisms that will cause spoilage and to block enzymes that reduce the quality of the berries. Molds, yeast and bacteria are present on fresh fruit and will grow quite rapidly under ordinary circumstances. This undesirable contamination can lead to deterioration and/or fermentation that is slowed by refrigeration and can be prevented by freezing or dehydration. However, if storage of the whole berries at room temperature is desirable, then these microbes need to be eliminated by heat. The canning jars obviously need to be sterilized by boiling immediately prior to adding the cooked berries. The heat also will degrade and inactive the proteinaceous enzymes that alter color, flavor and texture of the berries over time.

Whether to use fresh or blanched berries will depend on the berry. Once the fresh (and the fresher the better) firm berries are adequately rinsed of dirt and separated from extraneous matter such as plant and/or insect fragments, they can be placed in the sterilized jars and covered with boiling water or simmering juice extracted from cooked berries. Covering berries with their own juice instead of water helps them to keep their color and flavor. Firmer berries, such as blueberries, huckleberries, gooseberries, elderberries and currants, may first be placed in cheesecloth and dunked for 30 seconds of blanching in boiling water before canning (hot pack); this will soften them somewhat. Blackberries and raspberries should be placed in the jar raw (raw pack). (Strawberries are best frozen, not canned.) A hot syrup may be used to can fresh berries or a sweetener added to the hot cooked berries/juice/water, if necessary for sour berries like gooseberries.

To help prevent some immediate oxidative changes, crystalline ascorbic acid (vitamin C), citric acid or lemon juice can be added to the canning water or juice. The jars are transferred to the canner containing water that is hot (for fresh berries) or simmering (for blanched berries), and the water is brought to a rolling boil for the appropriate time, usually 15 or 20 minutes for pints or quarts, respectively. Jars are then carefully removed to cool, and as they do so the lids seal as the pressure inside is reduced. (A 'pop' of the lid is heard.)

The berries can be stored in a cool, dry place for up to a year. However, those that don't seal, and all when opened later to eat, need to be treated like fresh fruit and kept refrigerated. Specific canning instructions are readily available for various berries and should be followed to ensure appropriate procedures and enjoy success in making safe, nutritious, and delicious preparations. Canned berries are good to add to smoothies, on cold or cooked cereal, in pancakes or muffins, on yogurt or vanilla ice cream, or as a stand-alone snack or dessert.

Though glass jars are preferable for their inert quality of not interacting chemically with the berries, commercially canned berries are usually available in cans. These may be plasti-coated with bisphenol A to reduce chemical reactivity, but denting or a raised temperature increases the risk of leaching plastic or metal compounds into solution. Once opened, it is better to transfer berries bought in cans into another sealed container, preferably glass. In buying commercially canned fruit, aside from losing the control over choosing good quality berries for oneself, the label should be checked for undesirable additives and sweeteners, such as high fructose corn syrup.

Pure, unadulterated juice can likewise be home-canned by crushing food-quality berries and then simmering them over low heat. The pulp can be separated from the juice by allowing the juice to drip (not pressing with force) through cheesecloth in a colander while hot. The juice should be simmering hot when canned in sterilized (hot) glass jars.

DRIED BERRIES

Following the path of diminishing returns, after canned berries the next most preferable form is likely the air-dried berries. Though they contain the fiber lost in juices, beneficial phytochemicals can be greatly reduced, including total polyphenols based on dry weight, in addition to having lost the water from the fresh berry. The value of this water is not to be underestimated, as it is an inherent part of the living cellular matrix of the berry and maintains most of this complexity even after juicing. The water itself may provide a unique fingerprint of berry that is causing those in advanced research on the subject to marvel. However, that is a subject for a book of its own.

Drying is the oldest means of preserving berries. While this allowed them to be consumed later, often in other foods as flavoring and sweetening agent, the enzymatic conversions that occurred during the loss of the water over days time resulted in altered and diminished nutrient value. As the water loss occurs from the cells, cellular functions diminish and then cease, though the cell walls remain intact. Compounds are then bound together and to the structural fiber, making the digestion process to release these nutrients more difficult to accomplish, and thereby diminishing bioavailability.

Berries should be rinsed with cold water before drying; only solid intact berries should be used. They are placed on a tray in a single layer with space between berries. Drying techniques using an oven (with the door open a crack) or home food dehydrator will depend upon the nature of the berry. Since the berry skin, or cuticle, prevents water loss, solid berries may be sliced or punctured. Cranberries can be cut in half and will dry in 10-14 hours at about 55-60ºF (130-140ºC). Whole (unsliced) cranberries or blueberries will take about 24 hours at these temperatures, depending on the size. Higher temperatures reduce the time required but also the berry quality. Another way to reduce the time with whole cranberries or blueberries is to initially place them in a strainer in boiling water for 30-60 seconds, then doused in cold water to rapidly cool and cause the skin to crack, given moisture avenues of escape under the low heat of the oven or dehydrator. Results may be uneven. Raspberries can be dried whole if placed open-side down on a mesh drying screen, since the hollowness reduces the fleshy thickness. Solid segmented berries like blackberries need to be mashed and dried on a solid sheet.

Partial reconstitution of dried whole berries can be achieved by soaking them in water, but this does not reproduce the living fresh fruit with its matrix of soluble compounds. It is more similar to an extract of some of the berry components in solution within the membranes and cells of the berry "corpse", along with making the flavor and nutrients more readily available. The differences between a fresh grape and a soaked raisin remain manifold, even if soaking makes the raisin look more like a grape. Some berries rehydrate better than others. While *Vaccinium* speces like blueberries can regain some of their desirable plumpness, most *Rubus* species such as blackberries are too seedy to be enjoyed alone whether dried or rehydrated.

COMMERCIALLY BOTTLED BERRY JUICE

Actual pure juice sold commercially is often described as "fresh" juice, meaning that is was bottled when fresh, whereas most commercial "100%" juice is a juice concentrate (partially dehydrated) that has been reconstituted with filtered (tap) water. Sometimes, these reconstituted drinks are called pure juice, when they would be more accurately described as berry-flavored tap water or juice drinks.

Juice sold in brown glass bottles is much to be preferred over that sold in clear glass, due to chemical conversions from light exposure. Glass bottles are more preferable than plastic bottles or (plastic-coated) cans, since glass is inert and will not chemically interact with the juice.

In contrast, plastic can release compound into the juice, particularly when the juice and container are not refrigerated and especially when they are exposed to heat. Juice sold in cans likewise can react with the inside plastic-coating, or with a metal can when there is no plastic-coating. Since berries and their juice have an acid pH, the potential for interaction with an uncoated metal can is increased.

Juice sold in treated-paper cartons has the advantage of being opaque and blocking light, but again should be kept refrigerated to avoid heat-caused release of chemicals into the juice. In this regard, frozen juice concentrates sold in paper-based cylindrical cartons has the advantage of being kept frozen in opaque containers until the "juice" is consumed shortly after it is prepared, rather than sitting for extensive periods on store shelves. Always check the label for ingredients in any so-called juice or juice concentrate to be certain that there are no unfavorable additives. Commercial "juice cocktails", "juice drinks", and frozen juice drink concentrates are quite far from pure juice or simple water plus berry/fruit concentrates, since they are often diluted and have other additives, such as artificial coloring agents and sweeteners. These commercially sweetened juice drinks should be avoided, especially in large quantities and by children.

The disadvantages of commercial juice include those of fresh juice, that is, loss of fiber and nutrients bound to the fiber, along with some enzymatic chemical conversions inherent in the juicing process of mixing liquids from different cellular compartments in the berries. In addition, bottled or canned berry juices have been heated. This will block further enzymatic degradation, but the heating itself can degrade some nutrients and flavoring phytochemicals. The advantage of canned berry juice over canned berries is the reduction in bulk, but the loss of bulk is from the lost fiber and nutrients.

Another advantage of juice is that it can be consumed through a straw or otherwise drunk, which is appealing in certain situations, such as while travelling, and some physical conditions, including sore mouth, teeth, or throat. A problem inherent in juice-drinking is the overconsumption of sugar present in most fruit juice, in conjunction with its rapid absorption due to lack of fiber. One way to help avoid this tendency is by diluting bottled juice with sparkling water to produce a bubbly mixture that makes a suitable substitute for soda drinks, especially with children.

BERRY EXTRACTS

Unlike the other forms, the use of berries extracts for home consumption is not very common. Extracts are made by using a solvent to selectively withdraw certain soluble components from berries. The type of solvent used will determine which compounds are extracted, depending on their solubility. For instance, using a small amount of water to extract chopped dried berries by simmering, and then filtering out the pulp through cheesecloth, will remove the water-soluble constituents including sugars, anthocyanins, and associated compounds, suitable as a flavoring base. As such, an extract always contains only a part of the whole berry.

Soaking mashed berries in ethanol can extract some compounds not be removed in large amounts by water. The extract thus obtained can then be further extracted with a different solvent and separated to obtain a fraction that further concentrates particular components. This is repeated with other solvents for subfractions. The extraction process to obtain subfractions is often used in laboratory experiments to help identify the component(s) that has/have a particular activity. This more concentrated preparation can then be used in smaller doses that retain the desired bioactivity of these components. [Carried further, one isolated component can be purified for very a specific application. At the point of isolation of a single chemical, the complexity of a plant food product has been lost. When a pure substance is obtained, it is often destined for further pharmaceutical manipulation and/or synthesis, rather than being acquired for use through extraction.]

The American berries for which commercial extracts are most commonly found are the cranberry and chokeberry, since they are not commonly consumed as fresh berries due to sourness and astringency. The type of solvent used is determined by which components are most desired in the extract and what solvent is most efficient (and/or least expensive) for extracting them. Solid extracts featuring compounds that are not water soluble usually use organic solvents such as acetone or methanol that are toxic for human consumption. These solvents must be removed after making a liquid extract with them, resulting in a concentrated dry extract. In attempting to increase the ease of consumption and to reduce the quantity of consumption of berries or juice necessary for effectiveness, dry concentrated extracts are available in capsular form. Dry extracts are likely to be used for medicinal purposes and so are often standardized to contain a designated amount of specific constituents. It is important to note, however, that by concentrating certain compounds, other components with different beneficial activities will be lost in the process.

BERRY WINES

When an abundance of fresh berries is available, different means of home preserving are often utilized to provide a variety of consumable forms, based on culinary preferences and/or the ease of processing. In the case of berry wines, producing a fermented beverage that is both inebriating and nutritious is an enticing incentive to utilize this method, though it is more demanding than simply canning the fruit or juice. The berries used should be of good quality without bruises or mold. While wine-making kits are widely available for purchase, a general description of the process is given below.

Typically, home wine-making instructions describe procedures appropriate for 5 gallons (19-L) of wine production. This usually requires about 15 pounds of berries (fresh or frozen), but the appropriate amount depends on the berry and on individual preference for a strong- or light-flavored wine. Equipment should be sanitized by swishing or dousing with a stock solution of 4 teaspoons of potassium (meta)bisulfite mixed in 1/2 gallon of water (and saved for re-use). After crushing the berries with instruments that can be as simple as a 2 by 4 and a pail, sugar is added to the mix. The amount of alcohol produced depends on the amount of sugar available for fermentation, and even ripe berries are not very high in sugar. About 9 pounds of cane sugar is mixed in enough hot water to total 6 gallons when added to the mashed berries; after cooling, the sugar water is added to the mashed berries. To this is added 1/4 teaspoon potassium bisulfite, and the mixture is allowed to sit for a couple of days to eliminate wild yeast and bacteria. Then, a couple of grams of a tartaric, malic, and citric acid blend is added, the amount depending on the desired tartness. A little pectic enzyme should also be added according to label directions to help break down the pulp for greater clarity, and packaged wine yeast is stirred in for fermentation to occur in a temperature range between 65–75 °F (18–24 °C). This mixture is called "must".

The must is allowed to ferment for 5-7 days, stirring the pulp into the solution twice daily. The wine is then siphoned off into a 5-gallon glass carboy, leaving the berry pulp behind. The wine ferments another 10-15 days in the carboy until the bubbling nearly stops. The transfer of wine by siphoning from one container to another, called racking, is done every time the sediment at the bottom reaches 3/4 of an inch, to reduce off-flavors and cloudiness; aeration should be avoided during this process. After the third racking the fermentation can be nearly complete, and the wine begins to clear. Another 1/4 teaspoon of potassium bisulfite is added along with cane sugar water to sweeten to taste, if necessary or preferred. If this sugar water is used, then 2 1/2 teaspoons of potassium sorbate is also added to prevent further fermentation. This mixture is allowed to age for about 3 months in a cooler place, avoiding exposure to sunlight and oxygen. Before bottling, the bottles and corks are sterilized by rinsing with the strong stock potassium bisulfite solution. The bottles should be stored in a cool location around 45-50 °F (7-13 °C).

Commercial sources of berry wines are becoming more widely available. As with juice, wine should be consumed in moderate amounts, from 4-12 ounce daily depending on size, age, and gender, and those on medication should be aware of potential interactions. Similar to juice, it is beneficial to extend consumption by diluting the wine with sparling water according to taste, as a more nutritious alternative to wine coolers. For some strong-flavored homemade berry wines, diluting (and/or sweetening) may help enhance the flavor. In the case of wine, the alcohol content (around 11-12%) has replaced most of the sugar in the solution (except for what is added at the end). Whether a berry liquid contains sugar and/or alcohol, large amounts of these simple carbohydrates can have a detrimental impact in the short term and destructive effects in the long term if consumed daily. The way to optimize the nutritional value of berries is to ingest the whole fruit with its full nutrient matrix and fiber, preferably fresh or after being frozen but even when canned, as compared to only consuming the juice or wine.

BERRY PRESERVES OR JAMS

Firmer berries may be made into preserves, in which the intact fruit is suspended in a jelled syrup. Whether fresh or frozen, blueberries and blackberries, and especially softer berries like raspberries and strawberries, are usually crushed in sugar and made with into jams. The amount of sweetener depends on the type of berry used. White grape juice with stevia extract, juice concentrate, or honey can be used in place of granulated sugar; however, in these cases commercial universal (no-sugar) pectin should then be used. Some form of sweetener is needed to obtain the desirable gel-set and flavor. Specific recipes should be followed for each kind of berry and sweetener.

Both preserves and jams are jelled by using pectin, a soluble fiber found naturally in fruit, along with citric acid or lemon juice. Both preparations are canned in a manner similar to whole canned berries, though the filled cup-sized jars are boiled for only about 5 minutes in the canner. While both forms preserve the full content of cooked berries in a base of fruit fiber, the added sugar reduces the amount that should be consumed at any one time. Therefore, these forms only serve as condiments, not side dishes. In other words, they are consumed primarily for flavor, rather than for nutritional benefits. Jams and preserves are typically eaten with butter on plain or toasted bread or on pancakes or waffles. Small amounts can also be mixed with plain yogurt.

BERRY JELLIES OR SYRUPS

A jelly is made using clear juice and sugar with added pectin. Jellies are more firm than jams and do not contain fiber from the berries. Otherwise, they are prepared in much the same way as jams. Like jams and preserves, they are intended as condiments for adding flavor on bread, or even in tea, though they contain even less nutrients than the corresponding jams. Traditional use of parafin to seal the top of a jelly jar is no longer considered appropriate by those concerned with optimal preservation technique.

Juice from berries also function as a flavor for syrups. Blueberries, blackberries, raspberries, and strawberries are common sources of juices used in syrups. Syrups lack the pectin used in jellies that render jellies semisolid, so rather than being spread the syrups can be readily poured, whether over warm foods like pancakes and waffles or on cold desserts like ice cream. In either case, a syrup's flavor is used to enhance the food to which it is added, so it is also a condiment to be consumed in only small quantities due to its high sugar content.

Ordinary berry syrup begins with an equal number of cups of berries and sugar; low-sugar syrup uses a sugar content of about 3/4 the volume of berries, whereas a no-sugar syrup can use Stevia extract of around 1/4 the volume of berries. To begin, berries are crushed and cooked at full boil for 5-10 minutes with about 1 Tbs of lemon juice per 3 cups of berries. These cooked berries are strained through a collander or screen into a large saucepan; if a clear juice is desired, straining through cheesecloth or a jelly bag is preferable. The sugar is added to the filtered juice, brought to a boil, and simmered for one minute. Syrups can then be canned in jars like jellies or jams.

LIST OF ABBREVIATIONS

ABTS	2,2'-azino-bis(3-ethylbenzothiazoline-6-sulphonic acid
ACE	angiotensin I-converting enzyme
ADP	adenosine diphosphate
ALT	alanine transaminase
AST	aspartate transaminase
BHA	butylated hydroxyanisole
BHT	butylated hydroxytoluene
BUN	blood urea nitrogen
CAA	cellular antioxidant activity
CEACAM1	carcinoembryonic antigen-related cell adhesion molecule 1
CHD	coronary heart disease
CRP	C-reactive protein
CVD	cardiovascular disease
COX	cyclooxygenase
CYP	cytochrome P450
DNA	deoxyribonucleic acid
DPPH	2,2-diphenyl-1-picrylhydrazyl
dw	dry weight
EGCG	epigallocatechin gallate
ER	estrogen receptor
ERK	extracellular receptor kinase
FRAP	ferric reducing ability of plasma
fw	fresh weight
GAE	gallic acid equivalents
GGT	gamma-glutamyl transferase
GI	gastrointestinal
GST	glutathione S-transferase
HDL	high-density lipoprotein
HER2	human epidermal growth factor receptor 2
HR	hazard risk
HPFS/HPFUS	Health Professionals Follow-up Study
IC_{50}	half maximal inhibitory concentration
ICAM-1	intercellular adhesion molecule-1
IGF-1	insulin-like growth factor-1
IL	interleukin
iNOS	inducible nitric oxide synthase

INRs	international normalized ratio
JNK	c-Jun N-terminal kinase
LDL	low-density lipoprotein
L-NAME	L-NG-nitroarginine methyl ester
LOH	loss of heterozygosity
LOX	lipoxygenase
LT	leucotrienes
MAPK	mitogen-activated protein kinase
MDA	malondialdehyde
MI	myocardial infarction
MMPs	matrix metalloproteinases
mRNA	messenger ribonucleic acid
MRSA	methycillin-resistant *Staphylococcus aureus*
NDEA	N-nitrosodiethylamine
NF-κB	nuclear factor-kappa B
NHS I	first Nurses Health Study (1984-2008)
NHS II	2nd Nurses Health Study (1991-2007)
NMBA	N-nitrosomethylbenzylamine
NO	nitric oxide
NOS	nitric oxide synthase
NQO1	NAD(P)H:quinone oxidoreductase-1
NSAID	nonsteroidal anti-inflammatory drug
ODC	ornithine decarboxylase
OmG	O_6-methylguanine
ORAC	oxygen radical absorbance capacity
PACs	proanthocyanidins
PD	degree of polymerization
PG	prostaglandins
ppm	parts per million
PR	progesterone receptor
QR	NAD(P)H:quinone reductase

RNA	ribonucleic acid
ROS	reactive oxygen species
SBP	systolic blood pressure
SDH	sorbitol dehydrogenase
SGOT	serum glutamic-oxaloaceti transaminase
SGPT	serum glutamic-pyruvic transaminase
SPE	solid phase extracts
TAE	tannic acid equivalents
TBARS	thiobarbituric acid reactive substances
TEAC	Trolox equivalent antioxidant capacity
TNF-α	tumor necrosis factor-alpha
TPA	tumor promoter phorbol 12-myristate 13-acetate
UGT	UDP-glucuronosyltransferase
UTIs	urinary tract infections
UVB	ultraviolet-B
VCAM-1	vascular cell adhesion molecule-1
VEGF	vascular endothelial growth factor
VLDL	very low-density lipoprotein

Glyphs used to emphasize portions of the text.

References

I. Whole Fruits and Vegetables for Helping Prevent Chronic Diseases

1. Seeram NP. Berry fruits: compositional elements, biochemical activities, and the impact of their intake on human health, performance, and disease. *J. Agric. Food Chem.*, 56:627-9, 2008

2. Johnson EJ. The role of carotenoids in human health. *Nutr. Clin. Car.*, 5(2):56-65, 2002

3. Sluijs I, Beulens JWJ, Grobbee DE, et al. Dietary carotenoid intake is associated with lower prevalence of metabolic syndrome in middle-aged and elderly men. *J. Nutr.*, 139:987-992, 2009

4. Miller NJ, Ruiz-Larrea MB. Flavonoids and other plant phenols in the diet: their significance as antioxidants. *J. Nutr. Envir. Med.*, 12:39-51, 2002

5. Beekwilder J, Jonker H, Meesters P, et al. Antioxidants in raspberry: on-line analysis links antioxidant activity to a diversity of individual metabolites. *J. Agric. Food Chem.*, 53:3313-20, 2005

6. Seeram NP, Nair MG. Inhibition of lipid peroxidation and structure-activity-related studies of the dietary constituents anthocyanins, anthocyanidins, and catechins. *J. Agric. Food Chem.*, 50:5308-12, 2002

7. Pan M-H, Lai C-S, Ho C-T. Anti-inflammatory activity of natural dietary flavonoids. *Food Funct.*, 1:15-31, 2010

8. Hakkinen S, Auriola S. High-performance liquid chromatography with electrospray ionization mass spectrometry and diode array ultraviolet detection in the identification of flavonol aglycones and glycosides in berries. *J. Chromatogr.*, 829:91-100, 1998

9. Hakkinen SH, Karenlampi SO, Heinonen IM, et al. Content of the flavonols quercetin, myricetin, and kaempferol in 25 edible berries. *J. Agric. Food Chem.*, 47:2274-9, 1999

10. Amakura Y, Umino Y, Tsuji S, et al. Influence of jam processing on the radical scavenging activity and phenolic content in berries. *J. Agric. Food Chem.*, 48:6292-7, 2000

11. Vinson JA, Zubik L, Bose P, et al. Dried fruits: excellent in vitro and in vivo antioxidants. *J. Am. Coll. Nutr.*, 24(1):44-50, 2005

12. Wojdylo A, Figiel A, Oszmianski J. Effect of drying methods with the application of vacuum microwaves on the bioactive compounds,

color, and antioxidant activity of strawberry fruit. *J. Agric. Food Chem.,* 57:1337-1343, 2009

13. Wedick NM, Pan A, Cassidy A, et al. Dietary flavonoid intakes and risk of type 2 diabetes in US men and women. *Am. J. Clin. Nutr.,* 95(4):925-933, 2012

14. Lila MA. Impact of bioflavonoids from berryfruits on biomarkers of metabolic syndrome. *Funct. Foods Health Dis.,* 2:13-24, 2011

15. Cassidy A, O'Reilly EJ, Kay C, et al. Habitual intake of flavonoid subclasses and incident hypertension in adults. *Am. J. Clin. Nutr.,* 93:338-347, 2011

16. Joshipura KJ, Ascherio A, Manson JAE, et al. Fruit and vegetable intake in relation to risk of ischemic stroke. *JAMA,* 282(13):1233-39, 1999

17. Cassidy A, Mukamal KJ, Liu L, et al. High anthocyanin intake is associated with a reduced risk of myocardial infarction in young and middle-aged women. *Circulation,* 127:188-196, 2013

18. Mink PJ, Scrafford CG, Barraj LM, et al. Flavonoid intake and cardiovascular disease mortality: a prospective study in postmenopausal women. *Am. J. Clin. Nutr.,* 85:895-909, 2007

19. Dauchet L, Amouyel P, Hercberg S, et al. Fruit and vegetable consumption and risk of coronary heart disease: a meta-analysis of cohort studies. *J. Nutr.,* 136:2588-2593, 2006

20. Seeram NP. Berry fruits for cancer prevention: current status and future prospects. *J. Agric. Food Chem.,* 56:630-5, 2008

21. American Cancer Society website (medical review and revision: June 30, 2014; accessed Oct. 31, 2014)

    http://www.cancer.org/cancer/cancercauses/dietandphysicalactivity/diet-and-physical-activity

22. American Heart Association website (last reviewed February, 2014; accessed Oct. 31, 2014)

    http://www.heart.org/HEARTORG/GettingHealthy/NutritionCenter/HealthyEating/About-Fruits-and-Vegetables_UCM_302057_Article.jsp

23. Center for Disease Control and Prevention. Behavioral Risk Factor Surveillance System; Prevalence and trends data, nationwide (states, DC, and territories) - 2007 fruits and vegetables, http://apps.nccd.cdc.gov/brfss/list.asp?cat=FV&yr=2007&qkey=4415&state=All

24. Center for Disease Control and Prevention. Behavioral Risk Factor Surveillance System; Prevalence and trends data, nationwide (states, DC, and territories) - 2009 fruits and vegetables, http://apps.nccd.cdc.gov/brfss/list.asp?cat=FV&yr=2009&qkey=4415&state=All

25. Eaton DK, Kann L, Shanklin S, et al. Youth risk behavior surveillance - United States 2007. *Morb. Mortal. Week. Rep.,* 57(4):1-131, 2008

26. Eaton DK, Kann L, Shanklin S, et al. Youth risk behavior surveillance - United States 2009. *Morb. Mortal. Week. Rep.,* 59(SS-5), 2010

27. Knekt P, Kumpulainen J, Jarvinen R, et al. Flavonoid intake and risk of chronic diseases. *Am. J. Clin. Nutr.,* 76:560-568, 2002

28. Jennings A, Welch AA, Fairweather-Tait SJ, et al. Higher anthocyanin intake is associated with lower arterial stiffness and central blood pressure in women. *Am. J. Clin. Nutr.,* 96:781-788, 2012

29. Takachi R, Inoue M, Ishihara J, et al. Fruit and vegetable intake and risk of total cancer and cardiovascular disease – Japan Public Health Center-based prospective study. *Am. J. Epidemiol.,* 167:59-70, 2008

30. Rodriguez-Mateos A, Heiss C, Borges G, et al. Berry (poly)phenols and cardiovascular health. *J. Agric. Food Chem.,* 62(18):3842-3851, 2014

31. Vainio H, Weiderpass E. Fruit and vegetables in cancer prevention. *Nutr. Cancer,* 54(1):111-42, 2006

32. Negri E, LaVecchia C, Franceschi S, et al. Vegetable and fruit consumption and cancer risk. *Int. J. Cancer,* 48:350-4, 1991

33. Pavia M, Pileggi C, Nobile CGA, et al. Association between fruit and vegetable consumption and oral cancer: a meta-analysis of observational studies. *Am. J. Clin. Nutr.,* 83:1126-34, 2006

34. Albarracin SL, Stab B, Casas Z, et al. Effects of natural antioxidants in neurodegenerative disease. *Nutr. Neurosci.,* 15(1):1-7, 2012

35. Lau FC, Shukitt-Hale B, Joseph JA. The beneficial effects of fruit polyphenols on brain aging. *Neurobiol. Aging,* 26S:S128-S132, 2005

36. Joseph JA, Shukitt-Hale B, Casadesus G. Reversing the deleterious effects of aging on neuronal communication and behavior: beneficial properties of fruit polyphenolic compounds. *Am. J. Clin. Nutr.,* 81(suppl):313S-316S, 2005

37. Shukitt-Hale B, Lau FC, Joseph JA. Berry fruit supplementation and the aging brain. *J. Agric. Food Chem.,* 56:636-41, 2008

38. Barberger-Gateau P, Raffaitin C, Letenneur L, et al. Dietary patterns and risk of dementia. The three-city cohort study. *Neurology,* 69:1921-30, 2007

39. Cherniack EP. A berry thought-provoking idea: the potential role of plant polyphenols in the treatment of age-related cognitive disorders. *Br. J. Nutr.,* 108(5):794-800, 2012

40. Gao X, Cassidy A, Schwarzschild MA, et al. Habitual intake of dietary flavonoids and risk of Parkinson disease. *Neurol.,* 78:1138-1145, 2012

41. Wu X, Schauss AG. Mitigation of inflammation with foods. *J. Agric. Food Chem.*, 60:6703-6717, 2012

II. BERRIES AS NUTRIENT-DENSE FRUIT

1. Miller NJ, Ruiz-Larrea MB. Flavonoids and other plant phenols in the diet: their significance as antioxidants. *J. Nutr. Envir. Med.*, 12:39-51, 2002

2. Seeram NP, Nair MG. Inhibition of lipid peroxidation and structure-activity-related studies of the dietary constituents anthocyanins, anthocyanidins, and catechins. *J. Agric. Food Chem.*, 50:5308-12, 2002

3. Prior RL. Fruits and vegetables in the prevention of cellular oxidative damage. *Am. J. Clin. Nutr.*, 78(suppl):570S-8S, 2003

4. Seeram NP. Berry fruits: compositional elements, biochemical activities, and the impact of their intake on human health, performance, and disease. *J. Agric. Food Chem.*, 56:627-9, 2008

5. Seeram NP, Momin RA, Nair MG, et al. Cyclooxygenase inhibitory and antioxidant cyanidin glycosides in cherries and berries. *Phytomed.*, 8(5):362-9, 2001

6. Halvorsen BL, Carlsen MH, Phillips KM, et al. Content of redox-active compounds (ie, antioxidants) in foods consumed in the United States. *Am. J. Clin. Nutr.*, 84:95-135, 2006

7. Wu X, Beecher GR, Holden JM, et al. Lipophilic and hydrophilic antioxidant capacities of common foods in the United States. *J. Agric. Food Chem.*, 52:4026-37, 2004

8. Sun J, Chu Y-F, Wu X, et al. Antioxidant and antiproliferative activities of common fruit. *J. Agric. Food Chem.*, 50:7449-54, 2002

9. Moerman DE. *Native American Ethnobotany*, Timber Press, Portland, Ore., 1998

10. Berglund B, Bolsby CE. *The Edible Wild*, Charle's Scribners Sons, New York, NY, 1971

11. Angier B. *Field Guide to Medicinal Wild Plants*, Stackpole Books, Harrisburg, PA, 1978

12. Cook WH. *The Physiomedical Dispensatory* [1869]. Eclectic Medical Pub., Portland, OR, 1985

13. Felter HW, Lloyd JU. *King's American Dispensatory* [1898]. Eclectic Medical Pub., Portland, OR, 1983

14. Kuts-Cheraux AW. *Naturae Medicina and Naturopathic Dispensatory*, American Naturopathic Physicians and Surgeons Assoc., Des Moines, IA, 1953

15. Lust J. *The Herb Book*, Bantam Books, New York, NY, 1974

16. Bodel PT, Cotran R, Kass EH. Cranberry juice and the antibacterial action of hippuric acid. *J. Lab. Clin. Med.*, 54(6):881-888, 1959

III. HEATH FAMILY *VACCINIUM* BERRIES
BLUEBERRIES

1. Kalt W, Ryan DAJ, Duy JC, et al. Interspecific variation in anthocyanins, phenolics, and antioxidant capacity among genotypes of highbush and lowbush blueberries (*Vaccinium* section *canococcus* spp.). *J. Agric. Food Chem.*, 49:4761-4767, 2001

2. Prior RL, Cao G, Martin A, et al. Antioxidant capacity as influenced by total phenolic and anthocyanin content, maturity, and variety of *Vaccinium* species. *J. Agric. Food Chem.*, 46:2686-2693, 1998

3. Rodriguez-Mateos A, Cifuentes-Gomez T, Tabatabaee S, et al. Procyanidin, anthocyanin, and chlorogenic acid contents of highbush and lowbush blueberries. *J. Agric. Food Chem.*, 60:5772-5778, 2012

4. Rimando AM, Kalt W, Magee JB, et al. Resveratrol, pterostilbene, and piceatannol in *Vaccinium* berries. *J. Agric. Food Chem.*, 52:4713-9, 2004

5. Lyons MM, Yu C, Toma RB, et al. Resveratrol in raw and baked blueberries and bilberries. *J. Agric. Food Chem.*, 51:5867-5870, 2003

6. Rimando AM, Cuendet M, Desmarchelier C, et al. Cancer chemopreventive and antioxidant activities of pterostilbene, a nautrally occurring analogue of resveratrol. *J. Agric. Food Chem.*, 50:3453-3457, 2002

7. Wolfe KL, Rui HL. Cellular antioxidant activity (CAA) assay for assessing antioxidants, foods, and dietary supplements. *J. Agric. Food Chem.*, 55:8896-8907, 2007

8. Hakkinen SH, Karenlampi SO, Heinonen IM, et al. Content of the flavonols quercetin, myricetin, and kaempferol in 25 edible berries. *J. Agric. Food Chem.*, 47:2274-9, 1999

9. Kresty LA, Howell AB, Baird M. Cranberry proanthocyanidins induce apoptosis and inhibit acid-induced proliferation of human esophageal adenocarcinoma cells. *J. Agric. Food Chem.*, 56:676-80, 2008

10. Zheng W, Wang SY. Oxygen radical absorbing capacity of phenolics in blueberries, cranberries, chokeberries, and lingonberries. *J. Agric. Food Chem.*, 51:502-509, 2003

11. Muller D, Schantz M, Richling E. High performance liquid chromatography analysis of anthocyanins in bilberries (*Vaccinium myrtillus* L.), blueberries (*Vaccinium corymbosum* L.), and corresponding juices. *J. Food Sci.*, 77(4):C340-C335, 2012

12. Borges G, Degeneve A, Mullen W, et al. Identification of flavonoid and phenolic antioxidants in black currants, blueberries, raspberries, red currants, and cranberries. *J. Agric. Food Chem.*, 58:3901-3909, 2010

13. Srivastava A, Akoh CC, Fischer J, et al. Effect of anthocyanin fractions from selected cultivars of Georgia-grown blueberries on apoptosis and phase II enzymes. *J. Agric. Food Chem.*, 55:3180-3185, 2007

14. Pappas E, Schaich KM, Phytochemicals of cranberries and cranberry products: characterization, potential health effects, and processing stability. *Crit. Rev. Food Sci. Nutr.*, 49:741-781, 2009

15. Yousef GG, Brown AF, Funakoshi Y, et al. Efficient quantification of the health-relevant anthocyanin and phenolic acid profiles in commercial cultivars and breeding selections of blueberries (*Vaccinium* spp.). *J. Agric. Food Chem.*, 61:4806-4815, 2013

16. Blacker BC, Snyder SM, Eggett DL, et al. Consumption of blueberries with a high-carbohydrate, low-fat breakfast decreases postprandial serum markers of oxidation. *Br. J. Nutr.*, 109:1670-1677, 2013

17. Riso P, Klimis-Zacas D, Bo CD, et al. Effect of a wild blueberry (*Vaccinium angustifolium*) drink intervention on markers of oxidative stress, inflammation and endothelial function in humans with cardiovascular risk factors. *Eur. J. Nutr.*, 52:949-961, 2013

18. Wang Y-P, Cheng M-L, Zhang B-F, et al. Effect of blueberry on hepatic and immunological functions in mice. *Hepatobil. Pancreat. Dis. Int.*, 9(2):164-168, 2010

19. Smith MAL, Marley KA, Seigler D, et al. Bioactive properties of wild blueberry fruits. *J. Food Sci.*, 65(2):352-356, 2000

20. Prior RL, Gu L, Wu X, et al. Plasma antioxidant capacity changes following a meal as a measure of the ability of a food to alter in vivo antioxidant status. *J. Am. Coll. Nutrit.*, 26(2):170-181, 2007

21. Seeram NP, Nair MG. Inhibition of lipid peroxidation and structure-activity-related studies of the dietary constituents anthocyanins, anthocyanidins, and catechins. *J. Agric. Food Chem.*, 50:5308-12, 2002

22. Huang W-Y, Zhang H-C, Liu W-X, et al. Survey of antioxidant capacity and phenolic composition of blueberry, blackberry, and strawberry in Nanjing. *Biomed. & Biotechnol.*, 13(2):94-102, 2012

23. Nakajima J-I Tanaka I, Seo S, et al. LC/PDA/ESI-MS profiling and radical scavenging activity of anthocyanins in various berries. *J. Biomed. Biotech.*, 5:241-247, 2004

24. Pan M-H, Lai C-S, Ho C-T. Anti-inflammatory activity of natural dietary flavonoids. *Food Funct.*, 1:15-31, 2010

25. Seeram NP, Zhang Y, Nair MG. Inhibition of proliferation of human cancer cells and cyclooxygenase enzymes by anthocyanidins and catechins. *Nutr. Cancer*, 46(1):101-106, 2003

26. Vendrame S, Daugherty A, Kristo AS, et al. Wild blueberry (*Vaccinium angustifolium*) consumption improves inflammatory status in the obese Zucker rat model of the metabolic syndrome. *J. Nutr. Biochem.*, 24:1508-1512, 2013

27. Wu X, Cao G, Prior RL. Absorption and metabolism of anthocyanins in elderly women after consumption of elderberry or blueberry. *J. Nutr.*, 132:1865-1871, 2002

28. Mazza G, Kay CD, Cottrell T, et al. Absorption of anthocyanins from blueberries and serum antioxidant status in human subjects. *J. Agric. Food Chem.*, 50:7731-7737, 2002

29. Kalt W, Blumberg JB, McDonald JE, et al. Identification of anthocyanins in the liver, eye, and brain of blueberry-fed pigs. *J. Agric. Food Chem.*, 56:705-712, 2008

30. Kalt W, Hanneken A, Milbury P, et al. Recent research on polyphenolics in vision and eye health. *J. Agric. Food Chem.*, 58:4001-4007, 2010

31. Milbury PE, Kalt W. Xenobiotic metabolism and berry flavonoid transport across the blood-brain barrier. *J. Agric. Food Chem.*, 58:3950-3956, 2010

32. Andres-Lacueva C, Shukitt-Hale B, Galli RL, et al. Anthocyanins in aged blueberry-fed rats are found centrally and may enhance memory. *Nutrit. Neurosci.*, 8(2):111-120, 2005

33. Vendrame S, Guglielmetti S, Riso P, et al. Six-week consumption of a wild blueberry powder drink increased Bifidobacteria in the human gut. *J. Agric. Food Chem.*, 59:12815-12820, 2011

34. Russell WR, Labat A, Scobbie L, et al. Availability of blueberry phenolics for microbial metabolism in the colon and the potential inflammatory implications. *Mol. Nutr. Food Res.*, 51:726-731, 2007

35. Devore EE, Kang JH, Breteler MMB, et al. Dietary intakes of berries and flavonoids in relation to cognitive decline. *Ann. Neurol.*, 72:135-143, 2012

36. Krikorian R, Shidler MD, Nash TA, et al. Blueberry supplementation improves memory in older adults. *J. Agric. Food Chem.*, 58:3996-4000, 2010

37. Joseph JA, Denisova NA, Arendash G, et al. Blueberry supplementation enhances signaling and prevents behavior deficits in an Alzheimer disease model. *Nutrit. Neurosci.*, 6(3):153-162, 2003

38. Shukitt-Hale B, Lau FC, Carey AN, et al. Blueberry polyphenols attenuate kainic acid-induced decrements in cognition and alter inflammatory gene expression in rat hippocampus. *Nutrit. Neurosci.,* 11(4):172-181, 2008

39. Goyarzu P, Malin DH, Lau FC, et al. Blueberry supplemented diet: effects on object recognition memory and nuclear factor-kappa B levels in aged rats. *Nutrit. Neurosci.,* 7(2):75-83, 2004

40. Malin DH, Lee DR, Goyarzu P, et al. Short-term blueberry-enriched diet prevents and reverses object recognition memory loss in aging rats. *Nutrit.,* 27:338-342, 2011

41. Casadesus G, Shukitt-Hale B, Stellwagen HM, et al. Modulation of hippocampal plasticity and cognitive behavior by short-term blueberry supplementation in aged rats. *Nutrit. Neurosci.,* 7(5/6):309-316, 2004

42. Joseph JA, Shukitt-Hale B, Denisova NA, et al. Reversals of age-related declines in neuronal signal transduction, cognitive, and motor behavioral deficits with blueberry, spinach, or strawberry dietary supplementation. *J. Neurosci.,* 19(18):8114-8121, 1999

43. Shukitt-Hale B, Galli RL, Meterko V, et al. Dietary supplementation with fruit polyphenolics ameliorates age-related deficits in behavior and neuronal markers of inflammation and oxidative stress. *Age*, 27:49-57, 2005

44. Sweeney JI, Kalt W, Mackinnon SL, et al. Feeding rats diets enriched in lowbush blueberries for six weeks decreases ischemia-induced brain damage. *Nutrit. Neurosci.,* 5(6):427-431, 2002

45. Joseph JA, Fisher DR, Rimando AM, et al. Cellular and behavioral effects of stilbene reseveratrol analogues: implications for reducing the deleterious effects of aging. *J. Agric. Food Chem.,* 56:10544-10551, 2008

46. McGuire SO, Sortwell CE, Shukitt-Hale B, et al. Dietary supplementation with blueberry extract improves survival of transplanted dopamine neurons. *Nutr. Neurosci.,* 9(5/6):251-258, 2006

47. Papandreou MA, Tsachaki M, Efthimiopoulos S, et al. Cell-line specific protection by berry polyphenols against hydrogen peroxide challenge and lack of effect on metabolism of amyloid precurson protein. *Phytother. Res.,* 26(7):956-963, 2012

48. Basu A, Lyons TJ. Strawberries, blueberries, and cranberries in the metabolic syndrome: clinical perspectives. *J. Agric. Food Chem.,* 60(23):5687-5692, 2012

49. Cassidy A, O'Reilly EJ, Kay C, et al. Habitual intake of flavonoid subclasses and incident hypertension in adults. *Am. J. Clin. Nutr.,* 93:338-347, 2011

50. Wedick NM, Pan A, Cassidy A, et al. Dietary flavonoid intakes and risk of type 2 diabetes in US men and women. *Am. J. Clin. Nutr.*, 95(4):925-933, 2012

51. Muraki I, Imamura F, Manson JE, et al. Fruit consumption and risk of type 2 diabetes: results from three prospective longitudinal cohort studies. *Br. Med. J.*, 347:f5001[doi: 10.1136/bmj.f5001], 2013

52. Stull AJ, Cash KC, Johnson WD, et al. Bioactives in blueberries improve insulin sensitivity in obese, insulin-resistant men and women. *J. Nutr.*, 140:1764-1768, 2010

53. Basu A, Du M, Leyva MJ, et al. Blueberries decrease cardiovascular risk factors in obese men and women with metabolic syndrome. *J. Nutr.*, 140:1582-1587, 2010

54. Johnson SA, Figueroa A, Navaei N, et al. Daily blueberry consumption improves blood pressure and arterial stiffness in postmenopausal women with pre- and stage 1-hypertension: a randomized, double-blind, placebo-controlled clinical trial. *J. Acad. Nutr. Diet.*, 115(3):369-377, 2015

55. DeFuria J, Bennett G, Strissel KJ, et al. Dietary blueberry attenuates whole-body insulin resistance in high fat-fed mice by reducing adipocyte death and its inflammatory sequelae. *J. Nutr.*, 139:1510-1516, 2009

56. Kim H, Bartley GE, Rimando AM, et al. Hepatic gene expression related to lower plasma cholesterol in hamsters fed high-fat diets supplemented with blueberry peels and peel extract. *J. Agric. Food Chem.*, 58:3984-3991, 2010

57. Wu X, Kang J, Xie C, et al. Dietary blueberries attenuate atherosclerosis in apolipoprotein E-deficient mice by upregulating antioxidant enzyme expression. *J. Nutr.*, 140:1628-1632, 2010

58. Elks CM, Reed SC, Mariappan N, et al. A blueberry-enriched diet attenuates nephropathy in a rat model of hypertension via reduction in oxidative stress. *PLoS ONE*, 6(9):e24028(10 pp.), 2011

59. Rodriguez-Mateos A, Ishisaka A, Mawatari K, et al. Blueberry intervention improves vascular reactivity and lowers blood pressure in high-fat-, high-cholesterol-fed rats. *Br. J. Nutr.*, 109:1746-1754, 2013

60. Prior RL, Wu X, Gu L, et al. Whole berries versus berry anthocyanins: interactions with dietary fat levels in the C57BL/6J mouse model of obesity. *J. Agric. Food Chem.*, 56:647-653, 2008

61. Grace MH, Ribnicky DM, Kuhn P, et al. Hypoglycemic activity of a novel anthocyanin-rich formulation from lowbush blueberry, *Vaccinium angustifolium* Aiton. *Phytomed.*, 16(5):406-415, 2009

62. Martineau LC, Couture A, Spoor D, et al. Anti-diabetic properties of the Canadian lowbush blueberry *Vaccinium angustifolium* Ait. *Phytomed.*, 13:612-623, 2006

63. Iwao K, Kawai RT, Oda M, et al. Physicochemical interactions of metformin hydrochloride and glibenclamide with several health foods. *Yakugaku Zasshi*, 128(9):1341-1345, 2008

64. Ahmet I, Spangler E, Shukitt-Hale B, et al. Blueberry-enriched diet protects rat heart from ischemic damage. *PLoS ONE*, 4(6):e5954, 2009

65. Ahmet I, Spangler E, Shukitt-Hale B, et al. Survival and cardioprotective benefits of long-term blueberry enriched diet in dilated cardiomyopathy following myocardial infarction in rats. *PLoS ONE*, 4(11):e7975, 2009

66. Kalea AZ, Clark K, Schuschke DA, et al. Vascular reactivity is affected by dietary consumption of wild blueberries in the Sprague-Dawley rat. *J. Med. Food*, 12(1):21-28, 2009

67. Boateng J, Verghese M, Shackelford L, et al. Selected fruits reduce azoxymethane (AOM)-induced aberrant crypt foci (ACF) in Fisher 344 male rats. *Food Chem. Toxicol.*, 45:725-32, 2007

68. Stoner GD, Wang LS, Seguin C, et al. Multiple berry types prevent N-nitrosomethylbenzylamine-induced esophageal cancer in rats. *Pharm. Res.*, 27(6):1138-1145, 2010

69. Ravoori S, Vadhanam MV, Aqil F, et al. Inhibition of estrogen-mediated mammary tumorigenesis by blueberry and black raspberry. *J. Agric. Food Chem.*, 60(22):5547-5555, 2012

70. Aiyer HS, Gupta RC. Berries and ellagic acid prevent estrogen-induced mammary tumorigenesis by modulating enzymes of estrogen metabolism. *Cancer Prev. Res.*, 3(6):727-737, 2010

71. Adams LS, Kanaya N, Phung S, et al. Whole blueberry powder modulates the growth and metastasis of MDA-MB-231 triple negative breast tumors in nude mice. *J. Nutr.*, 141:1805-1812, 2011

72. Gordillo G, Fang H, Khanna S, et al. Oral administration of blueberry inhibits angiogenic tumor growth and enhances survival of mice with endothelial cell neoplasm. *Antiox. Redox Signal.*, 11(1):47-58, 2009

73. Suh N, Paul S, Hao X, et al. Pterostilbene, an active constituent of blueberries, suppresses aberrant crypt foci formation in the azoxymethane-induced colon carcinogenesis model in rats. *Clin. Cancer Res.*, 13(1):350-355, 2007

74. Rabin BM, Shukitt-Hale B, Joseph J, et al. Diet as a factor in behavioral radiation protection following exposure to heavy particles. *Grav. Space Biol.*, 18(2):71-78, 2005

75. Seeram NP, Adams LS, Zhang Y, et al. Blackberry, black raspberry, blueberry, cranberry, red raspberry, and strawberry extracts inhibit growth and stimulate apoptosis of human cancer cells in vitro. *J. Agric. Food Chem.*, 54:9329-9339, 2006

76. Yi W, Fischer J, Krewer G, et al. Phenolic compounds from blueberries can inhibit colon cancer cell proliferation and induce apoptosis. *J. Agric. Food Chem.*, 53:7320-7329, 2005

77. Yi W, Akoh CC, Fischer J, et al. Effects of phenolic compounds in blueberries and muscadine grapes on HepG2 cell viability and apoptosis. *Food Res. Int.*, 39:628-638, 2006

78. Schmidt BM, Erdman JW Jr, Lila MA. Differential effects of blueberry proanthocyanidins on androgen sensitive and insensitive human prostate cancer cell lines. *Cancer Lett.*, 231:240-246. 2006

79. Matchett MD, MacKinnon SL, Sweeney MI, et al. Inhibition of matrix metalloproteinase activity in DU145 human prostate cancer cells by flavonoids from lowbush blueberry (*Vaccinium angustifolium*): possible roles for protein kinase C and mitogen-activated protein-kinase-mediated events. *J. Nutrit. Biochem.*, 17:117-125, 2006

80. Ofek I, Goldhar J, Zafriri D, et al. Anti-*Escherichia coli* adhesin activity of cranberry and blueberry juices. *N. Eng. J. Med.*, 324(22)P1599, 1991

81. Bomser J, Madhavi DL, Singletary K, et al. *In vitro* anticancer activity of fruit extracts from *Vaccinium* species. *Planta Med.*, 62:212-216, 1996

82. McLeay Y, Barnes MJ, Mundel T, et al. Effect of New Zealand blueberry consumption on recovery from eccentric exercise-induced muscle damage. *J. Int. Soc. Sports Nutr.*, 9:19, 2012

83. Ramirez MR, Guterres L, Dickel OE, et al. Preliminary studies on the antinociceptive activity of *Vaccinium ashei* berry in experimental animal models. *J. Med. Food,* 13(2):336-342, 2010

84. Rabin BM, Shukitt-Hale B, Joseph J, et al. Diet as a factor in behavioral radiation protection following exposure to heavy particles. *Grav. Space Biol.*, 18(2):71-77, 2005

85. Schmidt BM, Howell AB, McEniry B, et al. Effective separation of potent antiproliferation and antiadhesion components from wild blueberry (*Vaccinium angustifolium* Ait.) fruits. *J. Agric. Food Chem.*, 52:6433-6442, 2004

86. Perkins-Veazie P. Blueberry, in Agric. Handbook No. 66: The commercial storage of fruits, vegetables, and florist and nursery stocks. Gross KC, Wang CY, Saltveit (eds.). U. S. Dep. Agric., Agric. Res. Serv., updated Aug., 2014

87. Fan L, Forney C, Song J, et al. Effect of hot water treatments on quality of highbush blueberries. *J. Food Sci.*, 73(6):M292-M297, 2008

88. Kalt W, Forney CF, Martin A, et al. Antioxidant capacity, vitamin C, phenolics, and anthocyanins after fresh storage of small fruits. *J. Agric. Food Chem.*, 47:4638-4644, 1999

89. Connor AM, Luby JJ, Hancock JF, et al. Changes in fruit antioxidant activity among blueberry cultivars during cold-temperature storage. *J. Agric. Food Chem.*, 50:893-898, 2002

90. Lohachoompol V, Srzednkicki G, Craske. The change of total anthocyanins in blueberries and their antioxidant effect after drying and freezing. *J. Biomed. Biotech.*, 2004(5):248-252, 2004

91. Reyes A, Evseev A, Mahn A, et al. Effect of operating conditions in freeze-drying on the nutritional properties of blueberries. *Int. J. Food Sci. Nutr.*, 62(3):303-306, 2011

92. Fracasseti D, Bo' CD, Simonetti P, et al. Effect of time and storage temperature on anthocyanin decay and antioxidant activity in wild blueberry (*Vaccinium angustifolium*) powder. *J. Agric. Food Chem.*, 61:2999-3005, 2013

93. Brownmiller C, Howard LR, Prior RL. Processing and storage effects on monomeric anthocyanins, percent polymeric color, and antioxidant capacity of processed blueberry products. *J. Food Sci.*, 73(5):H72-H79, 2008

94. Brown C, Howard LR, Prior RL. Processing and storage effects on procyanidin composition and concentration of processed blueberry products. *J. Agric. Food Chem.*, 57:1896-1902, 2009

95. Syamaladevi RM, Andrews PK, Davies NM, et al. Storage effects on anthocyanins, phenolics and antioxidant activity of thermally processed conventional and organic blueberries. *J. Sci. Food Agric.*, 92:916-924, 2012

96. Bo CD, Riso P, Brambilla A, et al. Blanching improves anthocyanin absorption from highbush blueberry (*Vaccinium corymbosum* L.) puree in healthy human volunteers: a pilot study. *J. Agric. Food Chem.*, 60:9298-9304, 2012

97. Rodriguez-Mateos A, Cifuentes-Gomex T, George TW, et al. Impact of cooking, proving, and baking on the (poly)phenol content of wild blueberry. *J. Agric. Food Chem.*, 62(18):3979-3986, 2014

98. Skrede G, Wrolstad RE, Durst RW. Changes in anthocyanins and polyphenolics during juice processing of highbush blueberries (*Vaccinium corymbosum* L.). *J. Food Sci.*, 65(2):357-364, 2000

99. Srivastava A, Akoh CC, Yi W, et al. Effect of storage conditions on the biological activity of phenolic compounds of blueberry extract packed in glass bottles. *J. Agric. Food Chem.*, 55:2705-2713, 2007

100. Yamamoto M, Yamaura K, Ishiwatari M, et al. Degradation index for quality evaluation of commercial dietary supplements of bilberry extract. *J. Food Sci.*, 78(3):S477-S483, 2013

101. Howard LR, Castrodale C, Brownmiller C, et al. Jam processing and storage effects on blueberry polyphenolics and antioxidant capacity. *J. Agric. Food Chem.*, 58:4022-4029, 2010

CRANBERRY

1. Leahy M, Speroni J, Starr M. Latest developments in cranberry health research. *Pharmaceut. Biol.*, 40(Suppl.):50-4, 2002

2. McKay DL, Blumberg JB. Cranberries (*Vaccinium macrocarpon*) and cardiovascular disease risk factors. *Nutrit. Rev.*, 65(11):490-502, 2007

3. Vinson JA, Bose P, Proch J, et al. Cranberries and cranberry products: powerful in vitro, ex vivo, and in vivo sources of antioxidants. *J. Agric. Food Chem.*, 56:5884-5891, 2008

4. Pappas E, Schaich KM. Phytochemicals of cranberries and cranberry products: characterization, potential health effects, and processing stability. *Crit. Rev. Food Sci. Nutr.*, 49:741-781, 2009

5. Valentova K, Steijskal D, Bednar P, et al. Biosafety, antioxidant status, and metabolites in urine after consumption of dried cranberry juice in healthy women: a pilot double-blind placebo-controlled trial. *J. Agric. Food Chem.*, 55:3217-3224, 2007

6. Kondo M, MacKinnon SL, Craft CC, et al. Ursolic acid and its esters: occurrence in cranberries and other *Vaccinium* fruit and effects on matrix metalloproteinase activity in DU145 prostate tumor cells. *J. Sci. Food Agric.*, 91:789-796, 2011

7. Viskelis P, Rubinskiene M, Jasutiene I, et al. Anthocyanins, antioxidative, and antimicrobial properties of American cranberry (*Vaccinium macrocarpon* Ait.) and their press cakes. *J. Food Sci.*, 74(2):C157-C161, 2009

8. McKay KD, Chen CYO, Zampariello CA, et al. Flavonoids and phenolic acids from cranberry juice are bioavailable and bioactive in healthy older adults. *Food Chem.*, 168:233-240, 2015

9. Kuzminski LN. Cranberry juice and urinary tract infections: Is there a beneficial relationship? *Nutr. Rev.*, 54(11):S87-90, 1996

10. Wing DA, Rumney PJ, Preslicka C, et al. Daily cranberry juice for the

prevention of asymptomatic bacteriuria in pregnancy: a randomized, controlled pilot study. *J. Urol.,* 180(4):1367-1372, 2008

11. Jepson RG, Craig JC. Cranberries for preventing urinary tract infections (Review). *Cochrane Database Syst. Rev.,* [doi:10.1002/14651858. CD001321.pub.4] 2008

12. Barbosa-Cesnik C, Brown MB, Buxton M, et al. Cranberry juice fails to prevent recurrent urinary tract infection: results from a randomized placebo-controlled trial. *Clin. Inf. Dis.,* 52:23-30, 2011

13. Bailey DT, Dalton C, Daugherty FJ, et al. Can a concentrated cranberry extract prevent recurrent urinary tract infections in women? A pilot study. *Phytomed.,* 14:237-41, 2007

14. Li M, Andrew MW, Wang J, et al. Effects of cranberry juice on pharmacokinetics of _-lactam antibiotics following oral administration. *Antimicrob. Agents Chemother.,* 53(7):2725-2732, 2009

15. Bohbot J-M. Results of a randomized, double-blind study on the prevention of recurrent cystitis with GynDelta®. *Gyn. Obster. J.,* Jan., 2007

16. Burleigh AE, Benck SM, McAchran SE, et al. Consumption of sweetened, dried cranberries may reduce urinary tract infection incidence in susceptible women - a modified observation study. *Nutr. J.,* 12(1):139(16 pp.), 2013

17. Takahashi S, Hamasuna R, Yasuda M, et al. A randomized clinical trial to evaluate the preventive effect of cranberry juice (UR65) for patients with recurrent urinary tract infection. *J. Infect. Chemother.,* 19:112-117, 2013

18. Ballester FS, Vidal VR, Alcina EL, et al. Cysticlean® a highly pac standardized content in the prevention of recurrent urinary tract infection: an observational, prospective cohort study. *BMC Urol.,* 13:28(6 pp.), 2013

19. McMurdo MET, Argo I, Phillips G, et al. Cranberry or trimethoprim for the prevention of recurrent urinary tract infections? A randomized controlled trial in older women. *J. Antimicrob. Chemother.,* 63(2):389-395, 2009

20. Vidlar A, Vostalova J, Ulrichova J, et al. The effectiveness of dried cranberries (*Vaccinium macrocarpon*) in men with lower urinary tract symptoms. *Br. J. Nutr.,* 104:1181-1189, 2010

21. Kessler T, Jansen B, Hesse A. Effect of blackcurrant-, cranberry- and plum juice consumption on risk factors, associated with kidney stone formation. *Eur. J. Clin. Nutr.,* 56:1020-1023, 2002

22. Gettman MT, Ogan K, Brinkley LJ, et al. Effect of cranberry juice consumption on urinary stone risk factors. *J. Urol.*, 174:590-594, 2005

23. Gotteland M, Andrews M, Toledo M, et al. Modulation of *Helicobacter pylori* colonization with cranberry juice and *Lactobacillus johnsonii* La1 in children. *Nutrition*, 24:421-426, 2008

24. Di Martino P, Agniel R, David K, et al. Reduction of *Escherichia coli* adherence to uroepithelial bladder cells after consumption of cranberry juice: a double-blind randomized placebo-controlled cross-over trial. *World J. Urol.*, 24:21-27, 2006

25. LaPlante KL, Sarkisian SA, Woodmansee S, et al. Effects of cranberry extracts on growth and biofilm production of *Eschericia coli* and *Staphylococcus* species. *Phytother. Res.*, 26(9):1371-1374, 2012

26. Zhang L, Ma J, Pan K, et al. Efficacy of cranberry juice on *Helicobacter pylori* infection: a double-blind, randomized placebo-controlled trial. *Helicobacter* 10(2): 139-145, 2004

27. Bonifait L, Grenier D. Cranberry polyphenols: potential benefits for dental caries and periodontal disease. *J. Can. Dent. Assoc.*, 76:a130, 2010

28. Babu J, Blair C, Jacob S, et al. Inhibition of *Streptococcus gordonii* metabolic activity in biofilm by cranberry juice high-molecular-weight component. *J. Biomed. Biotech.*, 2012:#590384, 7 pp., 2012

29. Hisano M, Bruschini H, Nicodemo AC, et al. Cranberries and lower urinary tract infection prevention. *Clinics,* 67(6):661-667, 2012

30. Nantz MP, Rowe CA, Muller C, et al. Consumption of cranberry polyphenols enhances human gd-T cell proliferation and reduces the number of symptoms associated with colds and influenza: a randomized, placebo-controlled intervention study. *Nutr. J.*, 2(1):161(15 pp.), 2013

31. Ruel G, Pomerleau S, Couture P, et al. Favourable impact of low-calorie cranberry juice consumption on plasma HDL-cholesterol concentrations in men. *Br. J. Nutr.*, 96:357-364, 2006

32. Ruel G, Pomerleau S, Couture P, et al. Plasma matrix metalloproteinase (MMP)-9 levels are reduced following low-calorie cranberry juice supplementation in men. *J. Am. Coll. Nutr.*, 28(6):694-701, 2009

33. Ruel G, Pomerleau S, Couture P, et al. Low-calorie cranberry juice supplementation reduces plasma oxidized LDL and cell adhesion molecule concentrations in men. *Br. J. Nutr.*, 9:352-359, 2008

34. Lee IT, Chan YC, Lin CW, et al. Effect of cranberry extracts on lipid profiles in subjects with Type 2 diabetes. *Diab. Med.*, 25:1473-1477, 2008

35. Shidfar F, Heydari I, Hajimiresmaiel SJ, et al. The effects of cranberry juice on serum glucose, apoB, apoA-I, Lp(a), and paraoxonase-1 activity in type 2 diabetic male patients. *J. Res. Med. Sci.,* 17(4):355-360, 2012

36. Dohadwala MM, Holbrook M, Hamburg NM, et al. Effects of cranberry juice consumption on vascular function in patients with coronary artery disease. *Am. J. Clin. Nutr.,* 93:934-940, 2011

37. Ruel G, Lapointe A, Pomerleau S, et al. Evidence that cranberry juice may improve augmentation index in overweight men. *Nutr. Res.,* 33:41-49, 2013

38. Duthie SJ, Jenkinson AM, Crozier A, et al. The effects of cranberry juice consumption on antioxidant status and biomarkers relating to heart disease and cancer in healthy human volunteers. *Eur. J. Nutr.,* 45:113-122, 2006

39. Simao TNC, Lozovoy MAB, Simao ANC, et al. Reduced-energy cranberry juice increases folic acid and adiponectin and reduces homocysteine and oxidative stress in patients with the metabolic syndrome. *Br. J. Nutr.,* 110:1885-1894, 2013

40. Basu A, Betts NM, Ortiz J, et al. Low-calorie cranberry juice decreases lipid oxidation and increases plasma antioxidant capacity in women with metabolic syndrome. *Nutr. Res.,* 31(3):190-196, 2011

41. Wilson T, Singh AP, Vorsa N, et al. Human glycemic response and phenolic content of unsweetened cranberry juice. *J. Med. Food,* 11(1):46-54, 2008

42. Wilson T, Luebke JL, Morcomb EF, et al. Glycemic responses to sweetened dried and raw cranberries in humans with type 2 diabetes. *J. Food Sci.,* 75(8):H218-H223, 2010

43. Khanal RC, Rogers TJ, Wilkes SE, et al. Effects of dietary consumption of cranberry powder on metabolic parameters in growing rats fed high fructose diets. *Food Funct.,* 1:116-123, 2010

44. Kim MJ, Ohn J, Kim JH, et al. Effects of freeze-dried cranberry powder on serum lipids and inflammatory markers in lipopolysaccharide treated rats fed an atherogenic diet. *Nutr. Res. Pract.,* 5(5):404-411, 2011

45. Kim MJ, Jung HN, Kim KN, et al. Effects of cranberry powder on serum lipid profiles and biomarkers of oxidative stress in rats fed an atherogenic diet. *Nutr. Res. Pract.,* 2(3):158-164, 2008

46. Shabrova EV, Tarnopolsky O, Singh AP, et al. Insights into the molecular mechanisms of the anti-atherogenic actions of flavonoids in normal and obese mice. *PLoS ONE,* 6(10):e24634, 2011

47. Duthie GG, Kyle JAM, Jenkinson AM, et al. Increased salicylate

concentrations in urine of human volunteers after consumption of cranberry juice. *J. Agric. Food Chem.*, 53:2897-900, 2005

48. Ferguson PJ, Kurowska EM, Freeman DJ, et al. In vivo inhibition of growth of human tumor lines by flavonoid fractions from cranberry extract. *Nutr. Cancer,* 56(1):86-94, 2006

49. De Angel RE, Smith SM, Glickman RD, et al. Antitumor effects of ursolic acid in a mouse model of postmenopausal breast cancer. *Nutr. Cancer,* 62(8):1074-1086, 2010

50. Prasain JK, Jones K, Moore R, et al. Effect of cranberry juice concentrate on chemically-induced urinary bladder cancers. *Oncol. Rep.,* 19(6):1565-1570, 2008

51. Seeram NP, Adams LS, Hardy ML, et al. Total cranberry extract versus its phytochemical constituents: antiproliferative and synergistic effects against human tumor cell lines. *J. Agric. Food Chem.,* 52:2512-2517, 2004

52. Chatelain K, Phippen S, McCabe J, et al. Cranberry and grape seed extracts inhibit the proliferative phenotype of oral squamous cell carcinomas. *Evid. Based Compl. Altern. Med.,* 2011:#467691 (12 pp.), 2011

53. Rimando AM, Kalt W, Magee JB, et al. Resveratrol, pterostilbene, and piceatannol in *Vaccinium* berries. *J. Agric. Food Chem.,* 52:4713-4719, 2004

54. Kresty LA, Howell AB, Baird M. Cranberry proanthocyanidins induce apoptosis and inhibit acid-induced proliferation of human esophageal adenocarcinoma cells. *J. Agric. Food Chem.,* 56:676-680, 2008

55. Kresty LA, Clarke J, Ezell K, et al. MicroRNA alterations in Barrett's esophagus, esophageal adenocarcinoma, and esophageal adenocarcinoma cell lines following cranberry extract treatment: insights for chemoprevention. *J. Carcinogen.,* 10:#34, 2011

56. Ferguson PJ, Kurowska E, Freeman DJ, et al. A flavonoid fraction from cranberry extract inhibits proliferation of human tumor cell lines. *J. Nutr.,* 134:1529-1535, 2004

57. Deziel B, MacPhee J, Patel K, et al. American cranberry (*Vaccinium macrocarpon*) extract affects human prostate cancer cell growth via cell cycle arrest by modulating expression of cell cycle regulators. *Food Funct.,* 3:556-564, 2012

58. Bomser J, Madhavi DL, Singletary K, et al. *In vitro* anticancer activity of fruit extracts from *Vaccinium* species. *Planta Med.,* 62:212-216, 1996

59. Neto CC. Cranberries: ripe for more cancer research? *J. Sci. Food Agric.,* 91:2303-2307, 2011

60. Neto CC. Cranberry and blueberry: evidence for protective effects against cancer and vascular diseases. *Mol. Nutr. Food Res.,* 51:652-664, 2007

61. Aschengrau A, Ozonoff D, Coogan P, et al. Cancer risk and residential proximity to cranberry cultivation in Massachusetts. *Am J. Pub. Health,* 86(9):1289-1296, 1996

62. Brody JG, Aschengrau A, McKelvery W, et al. Breast cancer risk and historical exposure to pesticides and wide-area applications assessed with GIS. *Environ. Health Perspec.,* 112(8):889-897, 2004

63. Rodriguez-Saona C, Vorsa N, Singh AP, et al. Tracing the history of plant traits under domestication in cranberries: potential consequences on anti-herbivore defences. *J. Exp. Bot.,* 62(8):2633-2644, 2011

64. Dugoua J-J, Seely D, Perri D, et al. Safety and efficacy of cranberry (*Vaccinium macrocarpon*) during pregnancy and lactation. *Can. J. Clin. Pharmacol.,* 15(1):e80-e86, 2008

65. Heitmann K, Nordeng H, Hoist L. Pregnancy outcome after use of cranberry in pregnancy – the Norwegian mother and child cohort study. *BMC Compl. Altern. Med.,* 13:345(12 pp.), 2013

66. Lilja JJ, Backman JT, Neuvonen PJ. Effects of daily ingestion of cranberry juice on the pharmacokinetics of warfarin, tizanidine, and midazolam – probes of CYP2C9, CYP1A2, and CYP3A4. *Clin. Pharmacol. Ther.,* 81(6):833-839, 2007

67. Ansell J, McDonough M, Zhao Y, et al. The absence of an interaction between warfarin and cranberry juice: a randomized, double-blind trial. *J. Clin. Pharmacol.,* 49:824-830, 2009

68. Bonetta A, Di Pierro F. Enteric-coated, highly standardized cranberry extract reduces risk of UTIs and urinary symptoms during radiotherapy for prostate carcinoma. *Cancer Manage. Res.,* 4:281-286, 2014

69. Hamilton K, Bennett NC, Purdie G, et al. Standarized cranberry capsules for radiation cystitis in prostate cancer patients in New Zealand: a randomized double blinded, placebo controlled pilot study. *Support. Care Cancer,* 23:95-102, 2015

IV. Rose Family *Rubus* and *Aronia* Berries
Black Raspberry

1. Dossett M, Lee J, Finn CE. Inheritance of phenological, vegetative, and fruit chemistry traits in black raspberry. *J. Amer. Soc. Hort. Sci.,* 133(3):408-417, 2008

2. Wada L, Ou B. Antioxidant activity and phenolic content of Oregon caneberries. *J. Agric. Food Chem.,* 50:3495-3500, 2002

3. Tulio AZ Jr, Reese RN, Wyzgoski FJ, et al. Cyanidin 3-rutinoside and cyanidin 3-xylosylrutinoside as primary phenolic antioxidants in black raspberry. *J. Agric. Food Chem.*, 56:1880-1888, 2008

4. Montrose DC, Horelik NA, Madigan JP, et al. Anti-inflammatory effects of freeze-dried black raspberry powder in ulcerative colitis. *Carcinogen.*, 32(3):343-350, 2011

5. Stoner GD, Chen T, Kresty LA, et al. Protection against esophageal cancer in rodents with lyophilized berries: potential mechanisms. *Nutr. Cancer*, 54(1):33-46, 2006

6. Stoner GD. Foodstuffs for preventing cancer: the preclinical and clinical develpment of berries. *Cancer Prev. Res.*, 2(3):187-194, 2009

7. Anonymous. Evaluation of ellagic acid content of Ohio berries - final report. *Ohio State University Extension Information*. no date

8. Daniel EM, Krupnick AS, Heur Y-H, et al. Extraction, stability, and quantitation of ellagic acid in various fruits and nuts. *J. Food Comp. Anal.*, 2(4):338-49, 1989

9. Parry J, Su L, Moore J, et al. Chemical compositions, antioxidant capacities, and antiproliferative activities of selected fruit seed flours. *J. Agric. Food Chem.*, 54:3773-3778, 2006

10. Parry J, Yu L. Fatty acid content and antioxidant properties of cold-pressed black raspberry seed oil and meal. *J. Food Sci.*, 69(3):189-193, 2004

11. Stoner GD, Sardo C, Apseloff G, et al. Pharmacokinetics of anthocyanins and ellagic acid in healthy volunteers fed freeze-dried black raspberries daily for 7 days. *J. Clin. Pharmacol.*, 45:1153-1164, 2005

12. Tian Q, Giusti MM, Stoner GD, et al. Urinary excretion of black raspberry (*Rubus occidentalis*) anthocyanins and their metabolites. *J. Agric. Food Chem.*, 54:1467-1472, 2006

13. Chen W, Wang D, Wang L, et al. Pharmacokinetics of protocatechuic acid in mouse and its quantification in human plasma using LC-tandem mass spectrometry. *J. Chromatogr. B Analyt. Technol. Biomed. Live Sci.*, 908:39-44, 2012

14. He J, Wallace TC, Keatley KE, et al. Stability of black raspberry anthocyanins in the digestive tract lumen and transport efficiency into gastric and small intestinal tissues in the rat. *J. Agric. Food Chem.*, 57:3141-3148, 2009

15. Wu X, Pittman HE III, Prior RL. Fate of anthocyanins and antioxidant capacity in contents of the gastrointestinal tract of weanling pigs following black raspberry consumption. *J. Agric. Food Chem.*,54:583-589, 2006

16. Khanal R, Howard LR, Prior RL. Urinary excretion of phenolic acids in rats fed cranberry, blueberry, or black raspberry powder. *J. Agric. Food Chem.*, 62:3987-3996, 2014

17. Zhang Z, Knobloch TJ, Seamon LG, et al. A black raspberry extract inhibits proliferation and regulates apoptosis in cervical cancer cells. *Gyn. Oncol.*, 123:401-406, 2011

18. Narayanan BA, Geoffroy O, Willingham MC, et al. p53/p21(WAF1/ CIP1) expression and its possible role in G1 arrest and apoptosis in ellagic acid treated cancer cells. *Cancer Lett.*, 136:215-21, 1999

19. Mallery SR, TOng M, Shumway BS, et al. Topical application of a mucoadhesive freeze-dried black raspberry gel induces clinical and histologic regression and reduces loss of heterozygosity events in premalignant oral intraepithelial lesions: results from a multicentered, placebo-controlled clinical trial. *Clin. Cancer Res.*, 20(7):1910-1924, 2014

20. Mallery SR, Zwick JC, Pei P, et al. Topical application of a bioadhesive black raspberry gel modulates gene expression and reduces cyclooxygensae 2 protein in human premalignant oral lesions. *Cancer Res.*, 68(12):4945-4957, 2008

21. Shumway BS, Kresty LS, Larsen PE, et al. Effects of a topically applied bioadhesive berry gel on loss of heterozygosity indices in premalignant oral lesions. *Clin. Cancer Res.*, 14(8):2421-2430, 2008

22. Mallery SR, Budendorf DE, Larsen MP, et al. Effects of human oral mucosal tissue, saliva, and oral microflora on intraoral metabolism and bioactivation of black raspberry anthocyanins. *Cancer Prev. Res.*, 4(8):1209-1221, 2011

23. Han C, Ding H, Casto B, et al. Inhibition of the growth of premalignant and malignant human oral cell lines by extracts and components of black raspberries. *Nutr. Cancer,* 51(2):207-217, 2005

24. Rodrigo KA, Rawal Y, Renner RJ, et al. Suppression of the tumorigenic phenotype in human oral squamous cell carcinoma cells by an ethanol extract derived from freeze-dried black raspberries. *Nutr. Cancer,* 54(1):58-68, 2006

25. Kresty LA, Frankel WL, Hammond CD, et al. Transitioning from preclinical to clinical chemopreventive assessments of lyophilized black raspberries: Interim results show berries modulate markers of oxidative stress in Barrett's esophagus patients. *Nutr. Cancer,* 54(1):148-156, 2006

26. Stoner GD, Aziz RM. Prevention and therapy of squamous cell carcinoma of the rodent esophagus using freeze-dried black raspberries. *Acta Pharmacol. Sin.*, 28(9):1422-1428, 2007

27. Kresty LA, Morse MA, Morgan C, et al. Chemoprevention of esophageal tumorigenesis by dietary adminstration of lyophilized black raspberries. *Cancer Res.*, 61:6112-6119, 2001

28. Chen T, Hwang H, Rose ME, et al. Chemopreventive properties of black raspberries in N-nitrosomethylbenzylamine-induced rat esophageal tumorigenesis: Down-regulation of cyclooxygenase-2, inducible nitric oxide synthase, and c-Jun. *Cancer Res.*, 66(5):2853-2859, 2006

29. Chen T, Rose ME, Hwang H, et al. Black raspberries inhibit N-nitrosomethylbenzylamine (NMBA)-induced angiogenesis in rat esophagus parallel to the suppression of COX-2 and iNOS. *Carcinogen.*, 27(11):2301-2307, 2006

30. Stoner GD, Dombkowski AA, Reen RK, et al. Carcinogen-altered genes in rat esophagus positively modulated to normal levels of expression by both black raspberries and phenylethyl isothiocyanate. *Cancer Res.*, 68:6460-6467, 2008

31. Lechner JF, Reen RK, Dombkowski AA, et al. Effects of a black raspberry diet on gene expression in the rat esophagus. *Nutr. Cancer,* 60(S1):61-69, 2008

32. Wang L-S, Dombkowski AA, Seguin C, et al. Mechanistic basis for the chemopreventive effects of black raspberries at a late stage of rat esophageal carcinogenesis. *Mol. Carcinogen.*, 50:291-300, 2011

33. Wang L-S, Hecht SS, Carmella SG, et al. Anthocyanins in black raspberries prevent esophageal tumors in rats. *Cancer Prev. Res. (Phila.),* 2(1):84-93, 2009

34. Barch DH, Fox CC. Selective inhibition of methybenzylnitrosamine-induced formation of esophageal O^6-methylguanine by dietary ellagic acid in rats. *Cancer Res.*, 48:7088-7092, 1988

35. Wang L-S, Hecht S, Carmella S, et al. Berry ellagitannins may not be sufficient for prevention of tumors in the rodent esophagus. *J. Agric. Food Chem.*, 58(7):3992-3995, 2010

36. Aiyer HS, Li Y, Liu QH, et al. Dietary freeze-dried black raspberry's effect on cellular antioxidant status during reflux-induced esophagitis in rats. *Nutrit.*, 27:182-187, 2011

37. Peiffer DS, Zimmerman NP, Wang L-S, et al. Chemoprevention of esophageal cancer with black raspberries, their component anthocyanins, and a major anthocyanin metabolite, protocatechuic acid. *Cancer Prev. Res.*, 7(6):574-584, 2014

38. Reen RK, Nines R, Stoner GD. Modulation of N-nitrosomethylbenzylamine metabolism by black raspberries in the esophagus and liver of Fischer 344 rats. *Nutr. Cancer,* 54(1):47-57, 2006

39. Zikri NN, Riedl KM, Wang L-S, et al. Black raspberry components inhibit proliferation, induce apoptosis and modulate gene expression in rat esophageal epithelial cells. *Nutr. Cancer,* 61(6):816-826, 2009

40. Wang L-S, Arnold M, Huang Y-W, et al. Modulation of genetic and epigenetic biomarkers of colorectal cancer in humans by black raspberries: a phase I pilot study. *Clin. Cancer Res.,* 17(3):598-610, 2011

41. Wang L-S, Kuo C-T, Cho S-J, et al. Black raspberry-derived anthocyanins demethylate tumor suppressor genes through the inhibition of DNMT1 and DNMT3B in colon cancer cells. *Nutr. Cancer,* 65(1):118-125, 2013

42. Mentor-Marcell RA, Bobe G, Sardo C, et al. Plasma cytokines as potential response indicators to dietary freeze-dried black raspberries in colorectal cancer patients. *Nutr. Cancer,* 64(6):820-825, 2012

43. Wang L-S, Young M, Juo C-T, et al. Metabolomic profiling reveals a protective modulation on fatty acid metabolism in colorectal cancer patients following consumption of freeze-dried black raspberries. *Am. Assoc. Cancer Res. Proc.,* Abs. 163, 2013

44. Harris GK, Gupta A, Nines RG, et al. Effects of lyophilized black raspberries on azoxymethane-induced colon cancer and 8-hydroxy-2'-deoxyguanosine levels in the Fischer 344 rat. *Nutr. Cancer,* 40(2):125-133, 2001

45. Bi X, Fang W, Wang L-S, et al. Black raspberries inhibit intestinal tumorigenesis in Apc1638+/- and Muc2-/- mouse models of colorectal cancer. *Cancer Prev. Res. (Phila.),* 3(11):1443-1450, 2010

46. Johnson JL, Bomser JA, Scheerens JC, et al. Effect of black raspberry (*Rubus occidentalis* L.) extract variation conditioned by cultivar, production site, and fruit maturity stage on colon cancer cell proliferation. *J. Agric. Food Chem.,* 59:1638-1645, 2011

47. Paudel L, Wyzgoski FJ, Giusti MM, et al. NMR-based metabolomic investigation of bioactivity of chemical constituents in black raspberry (*Rubus occidentalis* L.) fruit extracts. *J. Agric. Food Chem.,* 62:1989-1998, 2014

48. Aiyer HS, Gupta RC. Berries and ellagic acid prevent estrogen-induced mammary tumorigenesis by modulating enzymes of estrogen metabolism. *Cancer Prev. Res.,* 3(6):727-737, 2010

49. Ravoori S, Vadhanam MV, Aqil F, et al. Inhibition of estrogen-mediated mammary tumorigenesis by blueberry and black raspberry. *J. Agric. Food Chem.,* 60:5547-5555, 2012

50. Madhusoodhanan R, Natarajan M, Singh JVN, et al. Effect of black raspberry extract in inhibiting NFkB dependent radioprotection in human breast cancer cells. *Nutr. Cancer,* 62(1):93-104, 2010

51. Duncan FJ, Martin JR, Wulff BC, et al. Topical treatment with black raspberry extract reduces cutaneous UVB-induced carcinogenesis and inflammation. *Cancer Prev. Res.*, 2(7):665-672, 2009

52. Huang C, Zhang D, Li J, et al. Differential inhibition of UV-induced activation of NFkB and AP-1 by extracts from black raspberries, strawberries, and blueberries. *Nutr. Cancer,* 58(2):205-212, 2007

53. Liu Z, Schwimer J, Liu D, et al. Black raspberry extract and fractions contain angiogenesis inhibitors. *J. Agric. Food Chem.,* 53:3909-3915, 2005

54. Feng R, Ni H-M, Wang SY, et al. Cyanidin-3-rutinoside, a natural polyphenol antioxidant, selectively kills leukemic cells by induction of oxidative stress. *J. Biol. Chem.,* 282(18):13468-13476, 2007

55. Jeong HS, Hong SJ, Lee T-B, et al. Effects of black raspberry on lipid profiles and vascular endothelial function in patients with metabolic syndrome. *Phytother. Res.,* 28:1492-1498, 2014

56. Gu J, Ahn-Jarvis JH, Riedl KM, et al. Characterization of black raspberry functional food products for cancer prevention human clinical trials. *J. Agric. Food Chem.,* 62(18):3997-4006, 2014

57. Lee J. Marketplace analysis demonstrates quality control standards needed for black raspberry dietary supplements. *Plant Foods Hum Nutr.,* 69:161-167, 2014

58. Das M, Bicker DR, Mukhtar H. Effect of ellagic acid on hepatic and pulmonary xenobiotic mechanism in mice: studies on the mechanism of its anticarcinogenic action. *Carcinogen.,* 6(10):1409-1413, 1985

59. Ahn D, Putt D, Kresty L, et al. The effects of dietary ellagic acid on rat hepatic and esophageal mucosal cytochromes P450 and phase II enzymes. *Carcinogen.,* 17(4):821-828, 1996

60. Barch DH, Rundhaugen LM, Pillay NS. Ellagic acid induces transcription of the rat glutathione S-transferase-Ya gene. *Carcinogen.,* 16(3):665-8, 1995

61. Barch DH, Rundhaugen LM. Ellagic acid induces NAD(P)H:quinone reductase through activation of the antioxidant responsive element of the rat NAD(P)H:quinone reductase gene. *Carcinogen.,* 15(9):2065-8, 1994

62. Aiyer HS, Vadhanam MV, Stoyanova R, et al. Dietary berries and ellagic acid prevent oxidative DNA damage and modulate expression of DNA repair genes. *Int. J. Mol. Sci.,* 9:327-341, 2008

63. Xue H, Aziz RM, Sun N, et al. Inhibition of cellular transformation by berry extracts. *Carcinogen.,* 22(2):351-356, 2001

64. Maas JL, Galletta GJ, Stoner GD. Ellagic acid, an anticarcinogen in fruits, especially in strawberries: a review. *HortSci.,* 26(1):10-14, 1991

65. Devipriya N, Sudheer AR, Srinivasan M, et al. Effect of ellagic acid, a plant polyphenol, on fibrotic markers (MMPs and TIMPs) during alcohol-induced hepatotoxicity. *Toxicol. Mech. Meth.,* 17:349-356, 2007

66. Devipriya N, Sudheer AR, Menon VP. Dose-response effect of ellagic acid on circulatory antioxidants and lipids during alcohol-induced toxicity in exprimental rats. *Fund. Clin. Pharmacol.,* 21:621-630, 2007

67. Devipriya N, Sudheer AR, Vishwanathan P, et al. Modulatory potential of ellagic acid, a natural plant polyphenol on altered lipid profile and lipid peroxidation status during alcohol-induced toxicity: a pathohistological study. *J. Biochem. Mol. Toxicol.,* 22(2):101-112, 2008

BLACK CHOKEBERRY

1. Kokotkiewicz A, Jaremicz Z, Luczkiewicz M. *Aronia* plants: a review of traditional use, biological activites, and perspectives for modern medicine. *J. Med. Food,* 13(2):255-269, 2010

2. Denev PN, Kratchanov CG, Ciz M, et al. Bioavailability and antioxidant activity of black chokeberry (*Aronia melanocarpa*) polyphenols: in vitro and in vivo evidences and possible mechanisms of action: a review. *Compr. Rev. Food Sci. Food Safe.,* 11:471-489, 2012

3. Chrubasik C, Li G, Chrubasik S. The clinical effectiveness of chokeberry: a systematic review. *Phytother. Res.,* 24:1107-1114, 2010

4. Oszmianski J, Wojdylo A. *Aronia melanocarpa* phenolics and their antioxidant activity. *Eur. Food Res. Technol.,* 221:809-813, 2005

5. Kulling SE, Rawel HM. Chokeberry (*Aronia melanocarpa*) - a review on the characteristic components and potential health effects. *Planta Med.,* 74:1625-1634, 2008

6. Mikulic-Petkovsek M, Schmitzer V, Slatnar A, et al. Composition of sugars, organic acids, and total phenolics in 25 wild or cultivated berry speccies. *J. Food Sci.,* 77(10):C1064-C1070, 2012

7. Wu X, Gu L, Prior RL, et al. Characterization of anthocyanins and proanthocyanidins in some cultivars of *Ribes, Aronia*, and *Sambucus* and their antioxidant capacity. *J. Agric. Food Chem.,* 52:7846-7856, 2004

8. Hwang SJ, Yoon WB, Lee O-H, et al. Radical-scavenging-linked antioxidant activities of extracts from black chokeberry and blueberry cultivated in Korea. *Food Chem.,* 146:71-77, 2014

9. Nakajima J-I, Tanaka I, Seo S, et al. LC/PDA/ESI-MS profiling and radical scavenging activity of anthocyanins in various berries. *J. Biomed. Biotech.,* 5:241-247, 2004

10. Saruwatari A, Isshiki M, Tamura H. Inhibitory effects of various beverages on the sulfoconjugation of 17_-estradiol in human colon carcinoma Caco-2 cells. *Biol. Pharm. Bull.*, 31(11):2131-2136, 2008

11. Zheng W, Wang SY. Oxygen radical absorbing capacity of phenolics in blueberries, cranberries, chokeberries, and lingonberries. *J. Agric. Food Chem.*, 51:502-509, 2003

12. Benvenuti S, Pellati F, Melegari M, et al. Polyphenols, anthocyanins, ascorbic acid, and radical scavenging activity of *Rubus, Ribes,* and *Aronia. J. Food Sci.*, 69(3):164-169, 2004

13. Kahkonen MP, Hopia AI, Vuorela HJ, et al. Antioxidant activity of plant extracts containing phenolic compounds. *J. Agric. Food Chem.*, 47:3954-3962, 1999

14. Taheri R, Connolly BA, Brand MH, et al. Underutilized chokeberry (*Aronia melanocarpa, Aronia arbutifolia, Aronia prunifolia*) accessions are rich sources of anthocyanins, flavonoids, hydroxycinnamic acids, and proanthocyanidins. *J. Agric. Food Chem.*, 61:8581-8588, 2013

15. Jakobek L, Seruga M, Krivak P. The influence of interactions among phenolic compounds on the antiradical activity of chokeberries (*Aronia melanocarpa*). *Int. J. Food Sci. Nutr.*, 62(4):345-352, 2011

16. Sueiro L, Yousef GG, Seigler D, et al. Chemopreventive potential of flavonoid extracts from plantation-bred and wild *Aronia melanocarpa* (black chokeberry) fruits. *J. Food Sci.*, 71(8):C480-C488, 2006

17. Hudec J, Bakos D, Mravec D, et al. Content of phenolic compounds and free polyamines in black chokeberry (*Aronia melanocarpa*) after application of polyamine biosynthesis regulators. *J. Agric. Food Chem.*, 54:3625-3628, 2006

18. Jeppsson N. The effects of fertilizer rate on vegetative growth, yield and fruit quality, with special respect to pigments, in black chokeberry (*Aronia melanocarpa*) cv. 'Viking'. *Sci. Hort.*, 83:127-137, 2000

19. Valcheva-Kuzmanova S, Blagovic B, Valic S. Electron spin resonance measurement of radical scavenging activity of *Aronia melanocarpa* fruit juice. *Pharmacogn. Mag.*, 8(30):171-174, 2012

20. Wilkes K, Howard LR, Brownmiller C, et al. Changes in chokeberry (*Aronia melanocarpa* L.) polyphenols during juice processing and storage. *J. Agric. Food Chem.*, 62:4018-4025, 2014

21. Horszwald A, Julien H, Andlauer W. Characterisation of aronia powders obtained by different drying processes. *Food Chem.*, 141:2858-2863, 2013

22. Vlachojannis C, Zimmermann BF, Chrubasik-Hausmann S. Quantification of anthocyanins in elderberry and chokeberry dietary supplements. *Phytother. Res.,* 29(4):561-565, 2015

23. Symonowicz M, Sykula-Zajac A, Lodyga-Chruscinska E, et al. Evaluation of polyphenols and anthocyanins contents in black chockeberry [sic] - *Photinia melanocarpa* (Michx.) fruits extract. *Acta Polon. Pharm.,* 69(3):381-387, 2012

24. Wiczkowski W, Romaszko E, Piskula MK. Bioavailability of cyanidin glycosides from natural chokeberry (*Aronia melanocarpa*) juice with dietary-relevant dose of anthocyanins in humans. *J. Agric. Food Chem.,* 58:12130-12136, 2010

25. Lala G, Malik M, Zhao C, et al. Anthocyanin-rich extracts inhibit multiple biomarkers of colon cancer in rats. *Nutr. Cancer,* 54(1):84-93, 2006

26. Wu X, Pittman HE III, Mckay S, et al. Aglycones and sugar moieties alter anthocyanin absorption and metabolism after berry consumption in weanling pigs. *J. Nutr.,* 135:2417-2424, 2005

27. Stanisavljevic N, Samardzic J, Jankovic T, et al. Antioxidant and antiproliferative activity of chokeberry juice phenolics during in vitro simulated digestion in the presence of food matrix. *Food Chem.,* 175:516-522, 2015

28. Gumienna M, Lasik M, Czarnecki Z. Bioconversion of grape and chokeberry wine polyphenols during simulated gastrointestinal in vitro digestion. *Int. J. Food Sci. Nutr.,* 62(3):226-233, 2011

29. Pilaczynska-Szczesniak L, Skarpanska-Steinborn A, Deskur E, et al. The influence of chokeberry juice supplementation on the reduction of oxidative stress resulting from an incremental rowing ergometer exercise. *Int. J. Sport Nutr. Exerc. Metab.,* 15(1):48-58, 2005

30. Skarpanska-Stejnborn A, Basta P, Sadowska J, et al. Effect of supplementation with chokeberry juice on the inflammatory status and markers of iron metabolism in rowers. *J. Int. Soc. Sports Nutr.,* 11:48(10 pp.), 2014

31. Sonoda K, Aoi W, Iwata T, et al. Anthocyanin-rich *Aronia melanocarpa* extract improves body temperature maintenance in healthy women with a cold constitution. *SpringerPlus,* 2:626(5 pp.), 2013

32. Valcheva-Kuzmanova S, Marazova K, Krasnaliev I, et al. Effect of *Aronia melanocarpa* fruit juice on indomethacin-induced gastric mucosal damage and oxidative stress in rats. *Exp. Toxicol. Pathol.,* 56:385-392, 2005

33. Matsumoto M, Hara H, Chiji J, et al. Gastroprotective effect of red pigments in black chokeberry fruit (*Aronia melanocarpa* Elliot) on acute gastric hemorrhagic lesions in rats. *J. Agric. Food Chem.*, 52:2226-2229, 2004

34. Kujawska M, Ignatowicz E, Ewertowska M, et al. Protective effect of chokeberry on chemical-induced oxidative stress in rat. *Hum. Exp. Toxicol.*, 30(3):199-208, 2010

35. Valcheva-Kuzmanova S, Borisova P, Galunska B, et al. Hepatoprotective effect of the natural fruit juice from *Aronia melanocarpa* on carbon tetrachloride-induced acute liver damage in rats. *Exp. Toxicol. Pathol.*, 56:195-201, 2004

36. Kowalczyk E, Kopff A, Fijalkowski P, et al. Effect of anthocyanins on selected biochemical parameters in rats exposed to cadmium. *Acta Biochim. Pol.*, 50(2):543-548, 2003

37. Atanasova-Goranova VK, Dimova PI, Pevicharova GT. Effect of food products on endogenous generation of N-nitrosamines in rats. *Br. J. Nutr.*, 78(2):335-345, 1997

38. Valcheva-Kuzmanova S, Stavreva G, Dancheva V, et al. Effect of *Aronia melanocarpa* fruit juice on amiodarone-induced pneumotoxicity in rats. *Pharmacogn. Mag.*, 10(38):132-140, 2014

39. Francik R, Krosniak M, Sanocka I, et al. *Aronia melanocarpa* treatment and antioxidant status in selected tissues in Wistar rats. *BioMed. Research Int.*, 2014:#457085(9 pp.), 2014

40. Valcheva-Kuzmanova SV, Eftimov MT, Tashev RE, et al. Memory effects of *Aronia melanocarpa* fruit juice in a passive avoidance test in rats. *Folia Med.*, 56(3):199-203, 2014

41. Ohgami K, Ilieva I, Shiratori K, et al. Anti-inflammatory effects of aronia extract on rat endotoxin-induced uveitis. *Invest. Ophthalm. Vis. Sci.*, 46(1):275-281, 2005

42. Kedzierska M, Olas B, Wachowicz B, et al. Effects of the commercial extract of aronia on oxidative stress in blood platelets isolated from breast cancer patients after the surgery and various phases of the chemotherapy. *Fitoter.*, 83:310-317, 2012

43. Kedrierska M, Malinowska J, Kontek B, et al. Chemotherapy modulates the biological activity of breast cancer patients plasma: the protective properties of black chokeberry extract. *Food Chem. Toxicol.*, 53:126-132, 2013

44. Kedzierska M, Glowacki R, Czernek U, et al. Changes in plasma thiol levels induced by different phases of treatment in breast cancer; the

role of commercial extract from black chokeberry. *Mol. Cell. Biochem.*, 372:47-55, 2013

45. Olas B, Wachowicz B, Nowak P, et al. Studies on antioxidant properties of polyphenol-rich extract from berries of *Aronia melanocarpa* in blood platelets. *J. Physiol. Pharmacol.*, 59(4):823-835, 2008

46. Dietrich-Muszalska A, Kpka J, Kontek B. Polyphenols from berries of *Aronia melanocarpa* reduce the plasma lipid peroxidation induced by ziprasidone. *Schizo. Res. Treat.*, 2014:#602390(7 pp.), 2014

47. Valcheva-Kuzmanova SV, Beronova AB, Momekov GT. Protective effect of *Aronia melanocarpa* fruit juice in a model of cisplatin-induced cytotoxicity in vitro. *Folia Med.*, 55(3&4):76-79, 2013

48. Pool-Zobel BL, Bub A, Schroder N, et al. Anthocyanins are potent antioxidants in model systems but do not reduce endogenous oxidative DNA damage in human colon cells. *Eur. J. Nutr.*, 38:227-234, 1999

49. Braunlich M, Slimestad R, Wangensteen H, et al. Extracts, anthocyanins and procyanidins from *Aronia melanocarpa* as radical scavengers and enzyme inhibitors. *Nutrients*, 5663-678, 2013

50. Kahkonen MP, Heinonen M. Antioxidant activity of anthocyanins and their aglycons. *J. Agric. Food Chem.*, 51:628-633, 2003

51. Naruszewicz M, Laniewska I, Millo B, et al. Combination therapy of statin with flavonoids rich extract from chokeberry fruits enhanced reduction in cardiovascular risk markers in patients after myocardial infraction [sic] (MI). *Atheroscler.*, 194:e179-e184, 2007

52. Duchnowicz P, Nowicka A, Koter-Michalak M, et al. In vivo influence of extract from *Aronia melanocarpa* on the erythrocyte membranes in patients with hypercholesterolemia. *Med. Sci. Monit.*, 18(9):CR569-574, 2012

53. Poreba R, Skoczynska A, Gac P, et al. Drinking of chokeberry juice from the ecological farm Dzieciolowo and distensibility of brachial artery in men with mild hypercholesterolemia. *Ann. Agric. Environ. Med.*, 16:305-308, 2009

54. Skoczynska A, Jedrychowska I, Poreba R, et al. Influence of chokeberry juice on arterial blood pressure and lipid parameters in men with mild hypercholesterolemia. *Pharmacol. Rep.*, 59(suppl. 1):177-182, 2007

55. Sikora J, Broncel M, Markowicz, et al. Short-term supplementation with *Aronia melanocarpa* extract improves platelet aggregation, clotting, and fibrinolysis in patients with metabolic syndrome. *Eur. J. Nutr.*, 51:549-556, 2012

56. Broncel M, Kozirog M, Duchnowixz P, et al. *Aronia melanocarpa* extract reduces blood pressure, serum endothelin, lipid, and oxidative stress marker levels in patients with metabolic syndrome. *Med. Sci. Monit.,* 16(1):CR28-34, 2010

57. Sikora J, Broncel M, Mikiciuk-Olasik E. *Aronia melanocarpa* Elliot reduces the activity of angiotensin I-converting enzyme - in vitro and ex vivo studies. *Oxid. Med. Cell. Long.,* 2014:#739721(7 pp.), 2014

58. Valcheva-Kuzmanova S, Kuzmanov K, Mihova V, et al. Antihyperlipidemic effect of *Aronia melanocarpa* fruit juice in rats fed a high-cholesterol diet. *Plant Foods Hum. Nutr.,* 62:19-24, 2007

59. Jurgonski A, Juskiewicz J, Zdunczyk Z. Ingestion of black chokeberry fruit extract leads to intestinal and systemic changes in a rat model of prediabetes and hyperlipidemia. *Plant Food Hum. Nutr.,* 63:176-182, 2008

60. Qin B, Anderson RA. An extract of chokeberry attenuates weight gain and modulates insulin, adipogenic and inflammatory signalling pathways in epididymal adipose tissue of rats fed a fructose-rich diet. *Br. J. Nutr.,* 108:581-587, 2012

61. Kim B, Ku CS, Pham TX, et al. *Aronia melanocarpa* (chokeberry) polyphenol-rich extract improves antioxidant function and reduces total plasma cholesterol in apolipoprotein E knockout mice. *Nutri. Res.,* 33:406-413, 2013

62. Ciocoiu M, Badescu L, Miron A, et al. The involvement of a polyphenol-rich extract of black chokeberry in oxidative stress on experimental arterial hypertension. *Evid. Based Compl. Altern. Med.,* 2013:#912769(8 pp.), 2013

63. Bell DR, Gochenaur K. Direct vasoactive and vasoprotective properties of anthocyanin-rich extracts. *J. Appl. Physiol.,* 100:1164-1170, 2006

64. Zapolska-Downar D, Bryk D, Malecki M, et al. *Aronia melanocarpa* fruit extract exhibits anti-inflammatory activity in human aortic endothelial cells. *Eur. J. Nutr.,* 51:563-572, 2012

65. Kim B, Park Y, Wegner CJ, et al. Polyphenol-rich black chokeberry (*Aronia melanocarpa*) extract regulates the expression of genes critical for intestinal cholesterol flux in Caco-2 cells. *J. Nutrit. Biochem.,* 24:1564-1570, 2013

66. Ryszawa N, Kawczynska-Drozdz A, Pryjima J, et al. Effects of novel plant antioxidants on platelet superoxide production and aggregation in atherosclerosis. *J. Physiol. Pharmacol.,* 57:611-626, 2006

67. Luzak B, Golanski J, Rozalski M, et al. Extract from *Aronia melanocarpa* fruits potentiates the inhibition of platelet aggregation in the presence of endothelial cells. *Arch. Med. Sci.,* 6(2):141-144, 2010

68. Sikora J, Markowicz-Piasecka M, Broncel M, et al. Extract of *Aronia melanocarpa*-modified hemostasis: in vitro studies. *Eur. J. Nutr.,* 53:1493-1502, 2014

69. Bijak M, Bobrowski M, Borowiecka M, et al. Anticoagulant effect of polyphenols-rich extracts from black chokeberry and grape seeds. *Fitoter.,* 82:811-817, 2011

70. Bijak M, Saluk J, Ponczek MB, et al. Antithrombin effect of polyphenol-rich extracts from black chokeberry and grape seeds. *Phytother. Res.,* 27(1):71-76, 2013

71. Malinowska J, Babicz K, Olas B, et al. *Aronia melanocarpa* extract suppresses the biotoxicity of homocysteine and its metabolite on the hemostatic activity of fibrinogen and plasma. *Nutrit.,* 28:793-798, 2012

72. Bijak M, Saluk J, Antosik A, et al. *Aronia melanocarpa* as a protector against nitration of fibrinogen. *Int. J. Biol. Macromol.,* 55:264-268, 2013

73. Balansky R, Ganchev G, Iltcheva M, et al. Inhibition of lung tumor development by berry extracts in mice exposed to cigarette smoke. *Int. J. Cancer,* 131:1991-1997, 2012

74. Krajka-Kuzniak V, Szaefer H, Ignatowicz E, et al. Effect of chokeberry (*Aronia melanocarpa*) juice on the metabolic activation and detoxication of carcinogenic N-nitrosodiethylamine in rat liver. *J. Agric. Food Chem.,* 57:5071-5077, 2009

75. Szaefer H, Krajka-Kuzniak V, Ignatowicz E, et al. Chokeberry (*Aronia melanocarpa*) juice modulates 7,12-dimethylbenz[a]anthracene induced hepatic but not mammary gland phase I and II enzymes in female rats. *Environ. Toxicol. Pharmacol.,* 31:339-346, 2011

76. Thani NAA, Keshavarz S, Lwaleed BA, et al. Cytotoxicity of gemcitabine enhanced by polyphenolics from *Aronia melanocarpa* in pancreatic cancer cell line AsPC-1. *J. Clin. Pathol.,* 67(11):949-954, 2014

77. Thani NAA, Sallis B, Nuttall R, et al. Induction of apoptosis and reduction of MMP gene expression in the U373 cell line by polyphenolics in *Aronia melanocarpa* and by curcumin. *Oncol. Rep.,* 28:1435-1442, 2012

78. Malik M, Zhao C, Schoene N, et al. Anthocyanin-rich extract from *Aronia meoncarpa* E. induces a cell cycle block in colon cancer but not normal colonic cells. *Nutr. Cancer,* 46(2):186-196, 2003

79. Bermudez-Soto MJ, Larrosa M, Garcia-Cantalejo JM, et al. Up-regulation of tumor suppressor carcinoembryonic antigen-related cell adhesion molecule 1 in human colon cancer Caco-2 cells following repetitive exposure to dietary levels of a polyphenol-rich chokeberry juice. *J. Nutr. Biochem.,* 18:259-271, 2007

80. Rugina D, Sconta Z, Leopold L, et al. Antioxidant activities of chokeberry extracts and the cytotoxic action of their anthocyanin fraction on HeLa human cervical tumor cells. *J. Med. Food,* 15(8):700-706, 2012

81. Sharif T, Alhosin M, Auger C, et al. *Aronia melanocarpa* juice induces a redox-sensitive p73-related caspase 3-dependent apoptosis in human leukemia cells. *PLoS ONE,* 7(3):e32526, 2012

82. Gasiorowski K, Szyba K, Brokos B, et al. Antimutagenic activity of anthocyanins isolated from *Aronia melanocarpa* fruits. *Cancer Lett.,* 119:37-46, 1997

83. Handeland M, Grude N, Torp T, et al. Black chokeberry juice (*Aronia melanocarpa*) reduces incidences of urinary tract infection among nursing home residents in the long term - a pilot study. *Nutr. Res.,* 34:518-525, 2014

84. Park S, Kim JI, Lee I, et al. *Aronia melanocarpa* and its components demonstrate antiviral activity against influenza viruses. *Biochem. Biophys. Res. Comm.,* 440:14-19, 2013

85. Braunlich M, Okstad OA, Slimestad R, et al. Effects of *Aronia mealocarpa* constituents on biofilm formation of *Escherichia coli* and *Bacillus cereus. Molecules,* 18:14989-14999, 2013

86. Ho GTT, Braunlich M, Austarheim I, et al. Immunomodulating activity of *Aronia melanocarpa* polyphenols. *Int. J. Mol. Sci.,* 15:11626-11636, 2014

87. Strippoli S, Lorusso V, Albano A, et al. Herbal-drug interaction induced rhabdomyolysis in a liposarcoma patient receiving trabectedin. *BMC Compl. Altern. Med.,* 13:199(5 pp.), 2013

88. Li J, Deng Y, Yuan C, et al. Antioxidant and quinone reductase-inducing constituents of black chokeberry (*Aronia melanocarpa*) fruits. *J. Agric. Food Chem.,* 60:11551-11559, 2012

89. Braunlich M, Christensen H, Johannesen S, et al. In vitro inhibition of cytochrome P450 3A4 by *Aronia melanocarpa* constituents. *Plant Med.,* 79:137-141, 2013

About the Author

Francis Brinker, N.D., obtained his doctorate in 1981 at the National College of Naturopathic Medicine in Portland, Oregon. He then completed a postgraduate fellowship in botanical medicine at his alma mater and for four years served as a clinical and classroom instructor at NCNM. Afterward, he taught botanical medicine for seven years at the Southwest College of Naturopathic Medicine in Tempe, Arizona.

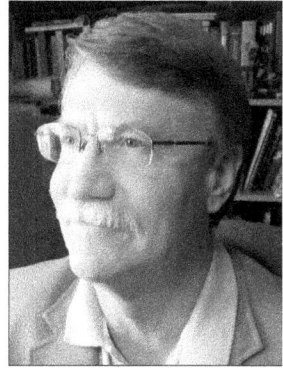

Dr. Brinker developed the initial botanical medicine sequence for the Program in Integrative Medicine at the University of Arizona. As a Clinical Assistant Professor there in the Department of Medicine, College of Medicine, he has been a member of the faculty since 2003.

Based on his extensive literature research of historic, scientific and medical publications, Francis Brinker has published many in-depth papers on botanical medicine. Some of his writings have been compiled in the *Eclectic Dispensatory of Botanical Therapeutics* vols. I & II (1989, 1995). The most recent editions of his books include *Formulas for Healthful Living* 2nd ed. (1998), *The Toxicology of Botanical Medicines* 3rd ed. (2000), *Complex Herbs – Complete Medicines* (2004), and *Herbal Contraindications and Drug Interactions plus Herbal Adjuncts with Medicines* 4th ed. (2010; Kindle 2013), all published by Eclectic Medical Publications.

Francis has been a regular reviewer for *American Herbal Pharmacopoeia* monographs since 1994 and *AHP* monograph co-author for Slippery Elm bark (2011), Blue Cohosh root (2012), and Boneset aerial parts (in process). He also acts as consulting editor for the American Botanical Council's *HerbClips*.

Dr. Brinker holds undergraduate degrees in human biology from Kansas Newman College and in biology from the University of Kansas, Phi Beta Kappa. Since 1986, he has worked as a consultant for Eclectic Institute, Inc., a natural products company that manufactures botanical supplements including liquid extracts and freeze-dried herbs, vegetables, fruits, and berries.

Works by Francis Brinker, N.D.

Books

Herbal Contraindications and Drug Interactions plus Herbal Adjuncts with Medicines, Fourth Edition (2010)

Complex Herbs – Complete Medicines (2004)

The Toxicology of Botanical Medicines, Third Edition. (2000)

Formulas for Healthful Living, Second Edition (1998)

The Eclectic Dispensatory of Botanical Therapeutics, vols. I & II (1989, 1995)

Selected Articles

"Potential for Interactions Between Dietary Supplements and Prescription Medications," (co-authored with Amit Sood, Richa Sood, Ravneet Mann, Laura L. Loehrer, Dietlind L. Wahner-Roedler) *The American Journal of Medicine*, 2008, vol. 121, no. 3, pp. 207-211.

"Wild yam – sorting out the species," *Journal of the American Herbalist Guild*, 2009, vol. 8, no. 2. pp. 3-13.

"Managing and Interpreting the Complexities of Botanical Research," *HerbalGram*, 2009, no. 82,
pp. 42-49.

"Prickly Pear as Food and Medicine," *Journal of Dietary Supplements*, 2009, vol. 6, no. 4, pp. 362-376.

"Boneset in dyspepsia and febrile infections," *Journal of the American Herbalist Guild*, 2010, vol. 9, no. 1, pp. 13-23.

"Echinacea Differences Matter: Traditional Uses of *Echinacea angustifolia* Root Extracts vs. Modern Clinical Trials with *Echinacea purpurea* Fresh Plant Extracts," *HerbalGram*, 2013, 97:46-57.

"Finally—a book that addresses one of the most important foods in our diet: berries. Brinker has written a readable, evidence-based guide for health professionals and anyone interested in learning more about the benefits of these amazing fruits."

Randy Horwitz, M.D., Ph.D.
Medical Director,
University of Arizona Center for Integrative Medicine

"*All American Berries* is beautifully written, accessible and compelling. It is filled with hundred's of research articles with concise, useful summaries. Dr. Brinker's blend of botany, pharmacognosy and naturopathic principles make this an essential text. The appendix is full of mouth-watering ways to consume a daily dose of berries. Berries are medicine!"

Louise N. Edwards, N.D., L.Ac.
Lecturer, Clinical Science, National University of Health Sciences
Adjunct Faculty, Bastyr University

"At the center of aging and many disease processes is inflammation and oxidation. Because of this, regular consumption of antioxidants is key to maintaining a long and vital life. In *All American Berries*, Dr. Brinker brings together the scientific evidence underscoring the health-promoting benefits of antioxidant-rich berries that are native to North America and are often overlooked as nutritional and botanical superstars for promoting health and longevity. "

Roy Upton, R.H., Dip.Ayu.
Executive Director, *American Herbal Pharmacopoeia*

"I didn't have any idea berries could be so interesting until I read what Dr. Brinker had to say about them! In this concise little book lies a wealth of information, copiously referenced, about the wide-ranging health benefits of berries, mainly blueberries, cranberries and black chokeberries, accompanied by the science behind why they are useful in so many health conditions from urinary tract infections to metabolic syndrome, cardiovascular disease to cancer. Dr. Brinker not only provides the health benefits of each type of berry, but identifies the constituents responsible for its tremendous healing and/or disease protective properties. Comparisons of different berry types show the health potentiating properties between them. There is even an appendix that reveals the advantages and limitations of different forms of storage and preparation. Reading it made me want to include different berries in their various forms at every meal to get all the health benefits they provide. Everyone interested in natural health needs a copy on their bookshelf for frequent reading and referencing."

James L. Wilson, D.C., N.D., Ph.D. in human nutrition
Author, *Adrenal Fatigue: The 21ˢᵗ Century Stress Syndrome*

"Dr. Brinker was one of my faculty during my integrative medicine fellowship. His text on drug-herb interactions was a key resource for safely using clinical botanicals. I greatly admire his vast knowledge and insight regarding nutrition and his ability to summarize the science in a pragmatic way. There are few foods as nutritionally powerful as berries. This text continues Dr. Brinker's tradition of combining the art with the science to empower us to improve the health of those we serve through one of nature's super foods. I highly recommend it."

David Rakel, M.D.
Founder and Director, University of Wisconsin Integrative Medicine Program
Associate Professor, Dept. of Family Medicine
University of Wisconsin School of Medicine and Public Health

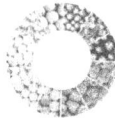